MW00803510

Neurocognitive Learning Therapy: Theory and Practice

Theodore Wasserman • Lori Drucker Wasserman

Neurocognitive Learning Therapy: Theory and Practice

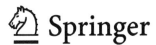 Springer

Theodore Wasserman
Wasserman and Drucker PA
Boca Raton, FL, USA

Lori Drucker Wasserman
Wasserman and Drucker PA
Boca Raton, FL, USA

ISBN 978-3-319-60848-8   ISBN 978-3-319-60849-5   (eBook)
DOI 10.1007/978-3-319-60849-5

Library of Congress Control Number: 2017944201

Printed on acid-free paper

This Springer imprint is published by Springer Nature
The registered company is Springer International Publishing AG
The registered company address is: Gewerbestrasse 11, 6330 Cham, Switzerland

Preface

When people find out that we wrote a book, the inevitable question is "How long did it take you to write that?" When one answers, the typical response is to tell the time from when you started writing, which in this case was somewhat over a year ago. When we started to think about the question in more detail, however, we realized that this book is the result of more than 25 years of clinical practice and discussion. Sometimes the discussions have been intense, and sometimes they have been outright heated, but in the end they represent a long period of intense research and daily interaction. That's not all we did. Along the way we raised three wonderful children, numerous dogs, the occasional cockatoo, and some unfortunately ill-fated fish.

What started out as a clinical observation, "How is it that kids with ADHD seem to pay attention to things that they like," has evolved into a fully articulated model of how people become mentally healthy and adaptive. It has also, by default, developed into a model of how people become mentally maladaptive and unhealthy. Based upon that model, we have developed a treatment paradigm, neurocognitive learning therapy. We believe it to be a unique "4th wave model" that is solidly based in neuroscience to achieve its explanatory power. Neurocognitive learning therapy is therefore both a theory of mental health and a method of treatment. When you understand the theory and incorporate the material into your clinical practice, you will become significantly more effective at ameliorating the difficulties that confront your clients.

Our discussions were not always between just the two of us. They often included neuropsychologists, neurologists, psychologists, and other professionals. We were fortunate to be able to present pieces of the model at conferences and receive feedback from attendees. We also received ongoing support from colleagues.

In particular, there were some people who were pivotal and without their contributions this book might not have reached fruition. We would like to thank Len Koziol for his belief in our work, his constant availability to provide feedback, and his willingness to provide an outlet for our initial work. Marci Fox was always supportive and amazingly positive. She always would say "Yes you can" when we were thinking no we can't. Finally, a big thanks to our senior editor Janice Stern and assistant editor Christina Tuballes for shepherding us through the process. They were ever supportive and always kind.

Boca Raton, FL, USA

Theodore Wasserman
Lori Drucker Wasserman

Introduction: A Model of Everything Therapeutic

As we developed neurocognitive learning therapy and therapy, the discussion inevitably turned to what kind of therapy NCLT represented. We suppose this is because humans, by definition, love to classify and categorize things in order to understand them better. It initially seemed logical that this new model had to be an iteration of some model that had come before. What became clear through the course of many discussions, however, is that NCLT is not a subclass of a prior model. While it is true that NCLT is built upon well-known therapeutic systems, the fusion of these systems represents a synthesis, or integration of the therapeutic process into a coherent whole, which may be unprecedented in the history of therapy. In this regard, it is a foundational model. It is a unifying model of all therapies, underpinned by an understanding of the brain-behavior relationship. This component is critical as it impacts the clinician's understanding of the etiology and maintenance of dysfunctional thoughts, feelings, and behavior patterns, which in turn affects how we proceed with our interventions. To be abundantly clear, rather than NCLT being an offshoot or embellishment of a currently existing therapy, it is the fusion of psychology and neuroscience, thereby creating the umbrella theory of therapy. In understanding the theory of NCLT, we better understand the totality of the person, allowing us to draw from various strategies, and apply the correct strategy to address the uniqueness of each client.

In order to advance the model, it will be necessary to look at other models of therapy and human development. We present them each with the intent of inclusion of the understanding of each position, and how clearly unified and integral each can be when looked at through the lens of NCLT.

The Development of NCLT

Given our backgrounds, we had immediately thought to ourselves that NCLT would be a new variant of cognitive behavior therapy (CBT). This initial assumption was in part determined by the use of cognitive disputation and reattribution techniques that occur regularly as part of NCLT practice. Cognitive behavior therapy emphasizes the primacy of cognition in mediating psychological disorder. It aims to alleviate distress by modifying cognitive content and process, realigning thinking and related emotion with reality.

At first, we were somewhat comfortable with placing NCLT within the cognitive behavioral framework, but the more we developed the model, the more the discussion turned to what NCLT had to say about the cognitive primacy vs affect primacy question. Primacy refers to how one initially responds to and processes information. As we reviewed our practices, coupled with neuroscience data, we realized that we had to incorporate the fact that in order to accommodate some of our clients, some of our intervention approaches were being spearheaded by the emotional, cognitive, or behavioral primacy factors which constituted a particular person's process patterns. People presented with different processing styles, and we were responding in kind. This led to the conclusion that we were in fact not traditional CBT therapists. We were not alone. In fact, for some CBT therapists, emotion has more recently become the dominant factor leading their therapeutic interventions. This is exemplified by the introduction of newer variants of cognitive therapy, such as DBT, which do include an emotive component, in recognition of the fact that better therapeutic gain was achieved for some by addressing their feeling states. Nonetheless, the question of primacy remains. This holds, despite the development of newer variations, because the question of primacy defines the intervention. That is, does a person become anxious first and ascribe a cognition to the emotion, or does this process happen in reverse. And how does this take account of more psychodynamic theories of, for example, object relations, which are of pre-linguistic origin? One's position, in part, determines which type of the abovementioned therapies one would engage in. We would likely all agree that a person enters the therapeutic process because they are in distress. But how does that distress come to be, how do they keep experiencing it, and how do we intervene become the questions we must ask. NCLT provides an answer with respect to primacy, and characteristically, it is not the answer most people expect.

Historical Divisions

Traditionally, there are two broad classes of primacy models: affective and cognitive. According to the older affective primacy models, affective information has priority, and its activation can precede identification of a linguistic category for a stimulus. That is, one reacts emotionally and then uses language to decipher the feeling state. This is often countered by cognitive primacy models, which asserts that a person must know what they are looking at before they can make an affective judgment about it.

Traditional Approaches Explained

Traditional affect (emotion) theorists contend that a person's emotional reaction to an event is the direct sequelae of either bodily states or neurophysiological processes. It is a thing to be experienced and does not have preconditions such as analysis or interpretation. Recently, affect theorists have bolstered their argument by noting that their view of an affective primacy, and affective state independence, is derived from a series of findings and phenomena, including the existence of neuroanatomical structures (and neural networks) dedicated to allowing for independent affective process. A related assumption in affective theories of emotion is that there exists a small set of basic emotions and that there are neurophysiological and anatomical substrates corresponding to the basic emotions. Psychologically, basic emotions are considered to be the primitive building blocks of other, sophisticated, non-basic emotions.

NCLT has a strong respect for human development. NCLT recognizes early neurophysiological arousal as a very necessary survival mechanism. For the practicing clinician, what needs to be discriminated is the relationship between these early fight or flight-based arousal responses and the later, partially linguistically labeled, complex emotions that confront us as part of a typical therapy practice. This relationship is explainable using life course and epigenetic models that are an integral part of NCLT. Suffice it to say at this point that the final emotional response is the product of a complex interaction between a constitutionally derived and environmentally experienced developmental process.

Cognitive Models

The affect position is countered by cognitive models that posit cognitive processes are essential to the experience of emotion. The cognitive perspective is based on the premise that emotional experience is contingent upon a person's appraisal and interpretation of the event or stimulus. This appraisal is often based on reinforcement history and or the individual's predisposition to interpret events in a particular manner. Ellis, in his rational emotive therapy A-B-C model, highlighted how the consequence (C) was the result of the belief (B), or appraisal, rather than the activating event (A) itself. Beck developed cognitive therapy highlighting dysfunctional thoughts as the etiology of dysfunctional feelings and behaviors.

Many people conclude that this means that cognitive therapists subscribe to the notion that thoughts cause feelings and that feelings cannot be created without thought. This is not entirely accurate, however. Cognitive behavior therapy posits that *modifying thought* has *primacy* when attempting to change many of the behaviors associated with mental dysfunction.

Neuropsychological Models

Neuropsychologists have focused on identifying various brain areas and systems that may mediate the experience of emotions. In this regard, neuropsychologists attempt to identify integrated brain networks involved in the expression of human emotion. The question of cognitive vs affect primacy has often produced mixed results, although we will later discuss newer research which supports the integrative model proposed by NCLT.

Cognitive and neuropsychological models usually posit that the genesis of emotional responses or affective states is dictated by the manner in which an individual ascribes meaning to the environment. In both models, emotions are produced and differentiated based on the perception of the situation or event as appraised by the individual. An added feature of neuropsychological models is that information processing or computational functions of integrated neural networks are hypothesized as the basis of all psychological processes, including emotion.

All of the above occurs in the context of the field not being able to agree upon how many emotions there are or what types of emotions exist. Some theorists still argue for a core of basic emotions that serve as the building blocks for all future emotions, and some people argue that there are as many emotions as there are individual people's responses to unique environmental situations. That is a lot of emotions.

Integrative Models

The situation remains confusing and largely unresolved and has led some to conclude that all of the research is indeterminant as regards primacy. Recent research has in fact indicated that there are elements of both cognitive and emotional primacy models in most situations. Others have taken a different approach and have tried to develop models that represent a fusion of what is known. These views frequently argue that cognitive networks that support information processing, and affect driven networks that support physiologically based emotional responses, initially exist independently of each other. They grow increasingly interdependent over time and reach the point where they are, in regard to emotion, one network indivisible. This most recent group of models, rather than seeking to solve the debate over Cognitive as opposed to affective primacy, posit that a more productive and accurate goal may be to determine the factors that cause affective information to have processing priority in some circumstances and semantic information in others. These models incorporate the truly integrated nature of the connectome as regards emotional respondency. They recognize that the same stimulus can activate different neurocognitive representations every time it is encountered. The specifics of the response is co-determined by the stimulus itself and the contexts in which it occurs.

NCLT and the Independence of Emotional States

NCLT considers the emotions encountered in therapy to be developed from cognitive labels, and the learned response tendencies associated with them are assigned to physiological changes resulting from the appraisal of threats, stress, or potential reward in the immediate environment. NCLT theory extends these appraisals to the contextually based cognitive labeling of an individual's physiological responses. Emotions are regarded as forms of cognitive appraisal evolved from experiences (initially flight or fight responses) and as states of action readiness related to the original pre-automatized appraisal. To answer the question regarding emotion's independence from cognition, it is important to look at this notion of action readiness.

Action Readiness

Action readiness essentially represents automated predictions of what the person is physiologically and cognitively primed to do (action tendency) in a given situation. In this view, emotions are grounded, primed, and stable activation patterns that have developed over time and, because of their high predictability, have become automatic. These predictions are continually updated by cognitive and bodily feedback and remain stable as long as the feedback remains as expected.

NCLT theory recognizes that primary emotional reactions are rooted in flight or fight responses that characterize the respondency of infants. For the more differentiated emotional responses (action tendencies) that develop later, an active cognitive labeling process is a critical part of development. The question regarding its potential to become independent from cognition is therefore changed and is framed by a different and often critical question: Is that active labeling process required every time that emotional response, which has already been primed, is triggered by a stimulus? For NCLT, and other action readiness models, the answer is that the active nature of the labeling process is not required every time one encounters that stimulus/event. To understand the reason that it isn't, one must understand automaticity. NCLT defines automaticity as a desired outcome of learning wherein a habitual behavior/response is elicited by environmental stimuli without conscious consideration of outcome. It is a desired outcome because humans have limited working memory and there is a need for a system that handles many mundane activities without contribution of higher order cognitive capacity. That system incorporates the activity rendering it automatic.

Automaticity implies that at some point in its development, an emotional response, if it is experienced enough, is able to be elicited by a stimulus without the benefit of the language-based or cognitive interpretation, which was critical in its formation. For example, think about a person who is afraid of spiders. When they see a spider, the emotional flight response is automatic. The individual does not have to go through a reasoning process. They are automatically afraid. Similarly, if a parent sees their child, they don't have to think about the fact that they love them. They just do. That is because the emotion and language labeling have been paired so many times that they are connected automatically, and the emotion is automatically produced as soon as the stimulus is presented. At that point, emotion is largely independent from cognition. This is a point we sought to make in our book, *Depathologizing Psychopathology* (2016). The goal of all learning, including emotional responding, is automaticity.

This is not to say that if you wanted to change the automatic emotional response you would not have to go back to the maintaining cognitive pairing as cognitive therapy suggests. You might very well have to, depending on the outcome you wanted. However, as classical conditioning models have demonstrated, you might not have to. In certain clinical situations, merely diminishing the undesirable emotional response may suffice.

The NCLT Answer

The more we learned, the more it became apparent that there was not a consensus as regards the primacy of cognition or emotion in the development of the emotional life of a human being. In fact, as we have seen, primacy may be the wrong question altogether in that there is increasing evidence that cognition and affect develop simultaneously, and cannot, and should not be picked apart. Primacy does remain a key question, however, as regards the treatment of problems associated with emotional regulation.

In its philosophical approach to the development and expression of emotion and its related behaviors, NCLT is very clearly in the integrative camp. As we have written elsewhere (Wasserman & Wasserman, 2016), NCLT posits that the networks that carry affective, physiologically based responses are integrated with cognitive appraisal networks to form a comprehensive and interdependent system for complex emotional and behavioral respondency. The end point in the generation of a complex emotion may, in fact, be an emotional and physiological response that is free of the cognitive elements that figured into its creation. This is because the goal of all human cognitive activity is the efficient use of working memory and the efficient creation of action potentials. NCLT's answer to the primacy question basically states that in the beginning of the creation of a complex emotional response the question of primacy is irrelevant, because all of the components, cognitive, physiological, and visceral, must be in place for the emotion to be created at all. The question does remain integral to treatment.

Primacy in Therapy

When it comes to the question of how to change emotional and related behavioral responses, it is vitally important to identify what is discussed and targeted in treatment.

Or so people continue to argue. Treatments differ. Some treatments target emotional responses first (tell me how you feel?), and other treatments target the cognitive appraisal of the situation (tell me how you think?). As regards the role of primacy in therapy, NCLT clearly postulates that the response to the question of primacy is situationally and/or person specific.

This situational specificity determines the NCLT therapist's response to the primacy question as regards the therapeutic endeavor. NCLT theory supports the concept that emotions may be regulated at any of five points in the emotion generative process: The therapist can choose when the individual identifies a particular situation as problematic, identifies a particular behavior as problematic within that situation, when they deploy their attention to a particular element of that situation, when they attempt to change a cognition associated with the situation, or if they want to change the emotional response to that situation. NCLT theory recognizes that different strategies have been postulated to achieve successful emotion regulation depending on the point of the process one wishes to highlight in the therapeutic discussion, and where in the process the best result can hypothetically be obtained. Techniques can run the gamut ranging from suppression, attentional control, distraction, and cognitive change to reappraisal. These techniques may include cognitive behavioral techniques, integrative techniques targeting the pairing of the emotional response and the related behavior, acceptance, relaxation, mindfulness, etc. NCLT asks you to remember that these techniques, many of which are successful and readily utilized, are techniques. NCLT is designed to help the practitioner understand the rationale for implementing any given technique at any given point. Therefore, more than a model of therapy, NCLT is a system of therapeutic interventions that incorporates and provides an empirically valid, etiological foundation for many of the known models of therapy.

Primacy, Recruitment, and Treatment of Disorders of Metal Health

The NCLT model suggests, in the context of disorders of mental health, that processes involved in emotional regulation are recruited during task performance. What this means is that there are learned contextual combinations of emotional, cognitive, and physiological responses that are a part of every disorder of mental health. For NCLT, therapy is considered a process of increasing the likelihood of the expression of adaptive behaviors, emotional responding, and thought processes and weakening or unlearning maladaptive ones. For NCLT, the therapy process goal is to eliminate maladaptive behaviors and thoughts which have become automatic and develop new adaptive behaviors and thoughts which will become automatic. In NCLT, therefore, the cognitive appraisal and the emotional response are components of an integrated whole, and primacy is relegated to an interesting question for intervention purposes. That is, an emotion, physiologic response, or thought can be clinically chosen, targeted by an empirically valid change technique selected by the clinician based upon its goodness of fit with the goal and processing style of the client, and the therapeutic result would be the same: new learning and a new set of responses.

Clearly then, there are situations where the discussion of cognitive appraisal is important, emotional appraisal is important, and developmental issues and automaticity are important. Just as clearly, the selection of an approach in the NCLT model does not therefore depend on the answer to the question of primacy per se, but rather recognizes the relative contribution of each of the above factors to the complexities of the individual, and relies on the identification of the target response, cognitive, emotional, or automatic visceral responding, the process of its development and maintenance, and the utilization of an empirically valid technique to change it. Within this foundational model, all prior models of therapy have a place. NCLT helps to explain why.

Reference

Wasserman, T., & Wasserman, L. (2016). *Depathologizing psychopathology*. New York: Springer.

Contents

Part I
NCLT Theory

Neurocognitive learning theory, as regards the development of mentally healthy behavior, is based on contributions from three branches of science: learning theory, small world hub models of cognitive processing, and epigenetics. In this first part, we will discuss the contributions of each of these to the overall model.

NCLT theory of treatment is based upon the above three branches with added consideration of the contribution of the science regarding reward valuation, automaticity, and memory reconsolidation. These will also be discussed in this part.

For neurocognitive learning theory, learning is defined as a process which includes emotion, cognition, and neurophysiology. Behavior is defined as the expression of these components.

Chapter 1
Introduction to Neurocognitive Learning Therapy

Neurocognitive learning therapy (NCLT) is a unifying therapeutic system which targets disorders of mental health. It is designed to work with, and make use of, our understanding of how the human brain processes and learns information while respecting the inclusion of developmental life span (or life course) issues and neurophysiology. It is, as a therapeutic intervention, unique in this regard. Some mental health therapies were developed in response to specific etiological hypotheses (psychoanalysis) or operant learning principles (applied behavior analysis). Others had no etiological basis at all, but relied on healing concepts such as self-actualization. With full respect for the complexities that make up human qualities, NCLT is based on information processing theory and models of integrated brain networks organized along small word hub principles. There is nothing else like it.

As we have demonstrated in our earlier book *Depathologizing Psychopathology* (Springer 2016), understanding that all learning, whatever the subject, issue, or person and emotional valence thereof, occurs over the same neural networks, and is subject to the same laws governing working memory allocation, attention, processing efficiency, memory, and expression and engagement, makes it possible to develop a set of principles that would facilitate learning in the therapeutic environment. How this facilitated learning occurs in an environment where an individual is seeking to address issues related to mental health (therapy), is at the core of NCLT.

In this book, we will demonstrate how the principles of learning and understanding of integrated brain networks can be made into a unique and comprehensive intervention for disorders of mental health.

NCLT Is a Unique, Integrative System

NCLT represents a unique system that does not fall neatly into any of the existing therapeutic disciplines simply because it is a comprehensive fusion of neurophysiology and learning principles. We posit that therapeutic principles that form the core

© Springer International Publishing AG 2017   3
T. Wasserman, L.D. Wasserman, *Neurocognitive Learning Therapy: Theory and Practice*, DOI 10.1007/978-3-319-60849-5_1

of NCLT actually underlie the functionality of every other therapeutic modality. Therefore, this common core both permits and explains the use of the other models within NCLT practice.

There is some evidence in the literature on the practice of psychotherapy for the existence of this common core. Ablon and Jones (2002), and others, demonstrated that therapeutic disciplines could be reliably distinguished on a rating scale meant to assess features of therapist activity specific to the respective treatments, but in practice, the results showed that treatments contained an equivalent degree of what had been termed "common facilitative conditions." In sum, the actual implementation of a form of treatment, in this case interpersonal therapy and cognitive behavior therapy, could not be distinguished by the actual process of treatment. Simply put, while the therapists claimed to be operating according to a differing set of principles, they were in fact practicing in a similar manner. Ablon and Jones (2002) indicated that a possible explanation for how the process of treatments with different brand names and different prescribed techniques can be so similar lies in the theoretical language used by adherents of different forms of psychotherapy. They conjectured that clinicians from different orientations may use very different terminology to describe psychological constructs and processes that are actually quite similar. Because of these differences in language and ways of conceptualizing, treatments may appear quite different on the surface. However, once we move beyond theory-specific language and examine what actually occurs during treatment sessions, treatments approaches in fact share many common features.

Common Core

Ablon and Jones (2002) go on to describe what the nature of this shared process might be. They indicate that the focus on content, rather than process, contributes to the appearance of large differences across these treatments. As an example, they indicate that the content of what a cognitive behavior therapist discusses with a client (dysfunctional attitudes or irrational beliefs) is often quite different from the content which an interpersonal psychotherapy therapist might focus (e.g., disruptions in personal relationships). The nature of the interaction between therapist and client in both systems is, however, often quite similar. A cognitive behavior therapist may coach or educate a patient about more effective ways of thinking (e.g., to not "catastrophize"), while an interpersonal psychotherapy therapist might teach a patient how to manage relationships with significant others more effectively. The content is different, but the nature of the interaction is similar.

From an NCLT perspective, it is critical to note that for both treatments they reviewed, a therapist assumes an active, instructive, and authoritative role, and teaches patients to think or conduct themselves differently. Both systems then encourage their clients to practice these new ways of thinking and behavior in everyday life. NCLT is focused on providing the tools to understand and operationalize the conduct of therapeutic practice. As such, it speaks about what is the functional core of all modalities of treatment. That functional core is learning. All treatment, all therapy, is about learning. No matter what you call it, self-actualization, spiritual awakening, cognitive redefinition, mindfulness, eliminating maladaptive ideas, coping statements or assertive training, what we were always talking about was replacing one set of emotions, ideas, or behavior with a more adaptive other set of emotions, ideas, and behavior. We were, whether we realized it or not, always talking about learning.

NCLT recognizes this reality that therapists, at least implicitly, do have an idea about how people learn and understand that specific things need to be accomplished in order to facilitate learning. By articulating and operationalizing this common core, or shared set of principles, NCLT may be the first therapeutic discipline that has the potential to effectively integrate all of the other disciplines into an empirically valid and scientifically testable, universal model of therapy.

The Process of Therapy

At their core then, all forms of therapy share a common goal consisting of a process designed to increase the likelihood of the expression of adaptive behaviors and thought processes, and to weaken or unlearn maladaptive ones. Therapy, in this perspective, is about the therapist imparting information and having the person use that information to change behavior and emotional response sets. All therapy represents a form of learning. NCLT is directly instructive in helping the client understand the process and principles involved. As in other forms of learning, we strive to produce learners who understand how they learn, and who can use that understanding to continually enhance and develop their knowledge and effectiveness. We teach strategies based upon learning principles, and we teach both strategies and learning principles directly.

Therapy is a process of taking previously maladaptive, automatic behaviors and thoughts, de-automatizing them, and creating new, adaptive, automatic behaviors and thoughts (responses) to life's various situations. Attaining ultimate success in terms of self-fulfillment, or realizing one's potential, would be in effect, a decision that an individual made when they were no longer engaging in identifiably maladaptive behavior. Therapy, therefore, is about learning.

Learning in therapy is no different from learning in any other context. All learning is governed by the same principles and rules. The practicing therapist and client's job is to select learning opportunities and design activities that will make learning adaptive behaviors and thoughts more efficient and effective.

NCLT Is a Model Based on Teaching

As you will come to know, NCLT is a directive and teaching oriented model, so more directive therapists might initially feel more at home with it than classically trained non-directive therapists would. Practitioners of classic and newer derivatives of cognitive behavior therapy will find a good deal of common ground with NCLT practice in that NCLT does consider cognitions and emotions as learned behavior, and therefore modifiable by predictable learning techniques. NCLT differs from cognitive therapy in the important area of primacy. In NCLT, either emotional or cognitive responses can be primary as a result of context and ultimately, automaticity.

NCLT Respects What Is Known About the Conduct of a Therapist

The principles that embody NCLT practice are meant to enhance what we know about the value of the therapeutic relationship. Research has clearly indicated that a positive therapeutic relation is a key variable in the success of treatment. NCLT therapists acknowledge that while the creation of a supportive therapeutic relationship is an important attribute of any therapeutic interaction it, by itself, is not sufficient to insure the effectiveness of the relationship between a therapist and a client. There is some research evidence to support the idea that the therapeutic relationship is, by itself, not sufficient to produce change. Wampol (2015) reviewed research that indicated that there were three pathways of a contextual therapeutic change model that should be included as part of any therapeutic change model. These were the supportive therapeutic alliance, the creation of expectations through the explanation of the disorder and the treatment involved, and the enactment of health promoting actions. There is even some evidence in fact that the rating of a positive relationship in therapy by itself may represent a problem in the process of change. This is because a rating of a positive therapist client relationship was directly related to the number of emotional responses that the client does not share with their therapist (Regan & Hill, 1992).

NCLT includes these three components and integral processes in the therapeutic endeavor. In addition NCLT relies on the therapist understanding the constructs behind the presenting problems and having the tools to address them.

A positive therapist-client relationship in NCLT practice can be considered a desirable precondition to therapy. NCLT therapists, however, recognize that liking each other is not the goal of therapy. Clients may seek to please a therapist, and might describe the relationship as positive, even though nothing with respect to therapeutic goals has in fact changed. In fact, while a relationship might be positive, as evidenced by the client's positive regard of the therapist and vice versa, there exists the possibility that, within such a context, the client may in fact not be learning or understanding anything. NCLT is designed to help the therapist know what to do after that relationship has been established. NCLT is designed to be instructive and impart active learning so that the therapeutic process does not rely solely on a positive relationship, but includes value and is seen as effective.

Effectiveness is defined in NCLT practice as making measureable progress towards the specific goals that were developed for the treatment of the referral issues. What is most important is that the therapist use their judgment to understand where in the development of, and capacity of the development of ideas and concepts the client is, so that information can be presented that is understandable, accessible, and useable by the client. The therapist must understand how certain constructs are developed, and then be able to guide the client on a predictable path to the healthy development of those constructs.

The Core Principles of NCLT

Semantics

A basic premise of NCLT is that therapy is about learning. By whatever process utilized to develop this learning, therapy consists of taking a previously learned set of maladaptive beliefs and behaviors and replacing them with adaptive beliefs and behaviors. It is important to note that "adaptive behavior" in NCLT encompasses all of the facets of human functioning, not just strictly behaviors. These maladaptive beliefs and behaviors may be conscious (readily identifiable by the client), or highly automatized (unconscious and therefore not readily explicit to the client). Whatever the descriptions of the acquisition process and the therapeutic process used by the particular school of therapeutic thought, the goal of all therapeutic systems is to learn and express adaptive behavior. Elucidating this goal is not always a readily available skill for the client. The following is paraphrased from online therapy message boards and chat lists "I hate this question! (Talking about the question "What is your goal in therapy?") I can NEVER answer it when (a therapist asks)." "I usually say something like "I don't know what I want to change or what the end goal is" or "All I do know is that I don't want things to be like this forever."" I guess I will know therapy is at end when I am able to deal with life effectively and be able to form healthy relationships on my own." "To not let the past rule the future I suppose." At the core clients wish to feel and act differently and more successfully."

The best way to understand NCLT is to understand its core principles. NCLT really has three sets of principles that govern its operation. The first set of principles govern the conduct of the therapist and the expectations for the clients. The second set of principles involve how people learn information. The third set of principles discuss the operation of small world hub network models. The first set of principles will be reviewed here while the learning and neurophysiology principles will be discussed in Chap. 2.

1. **The therapist must focus on the client and how they will incorporate and utilize new knowledge.**

It is important to understand that, for a variety of reasons, all information is not useable all the time. There are preconditions that must be met before new information is accessible and usable by the client.

New Information Must Be at Odds with Existing Information

Both Piaget (1977) and Vygotsky (1934/1986) agree that the process of cognitive and related emotional change are initiated by a cognitive conflict of sorts that occurs when an individual realizes a new idea does not align with his current thinking or prior knowledge. Cognitive therapists are adept in purposefully creating these conflicts. NCLT posits that for therapy to be successful it is necessary for this moment of conflict to be purposeful, explicit, and clearly expected by the client to occur as part of therapy. The client must understand that the purposeful challenges to the status quo emotionally and behaviorally will be made. For that to occur, the client must first be cognizant and able to identify the components of a current schema surrounding the construct, and recognize that the new idea or fact is discordant with the information already held. In other words, it is a necessary precondition that the individual recognize that the new information belongs to a certain class of information that does not exactly correspond with what is already known about that class but has the potential to inform and modify the class. NCLT recognizes that when this moment of conflict occurs, an individual will seek out answers in order to align their thinking and resolve the conflict.

New Information Can't Be Too Challenging or It Will Be Rejected

Piaget terms this conflict between what is known and what is new as the "just right challenge" meaning that the new information was just difficult and challenging enough to disturb an individual's current conceptualization of how a certain class of things are. A goal in NCLT treatment is to cause changes in the target concept that to lead to a new understanding and expansion of the concept. Information that is too discordant with the existing information or represents very significant differences between what is known and what is new will represent too difficult a challenge for an individual will be rejected.

NCLT recognizes that it is critically important that both the therapist and the client examine the new information in relation to what is known, and discuss how it might be used to impact the target behavior. This is an active and ongoing discussion between therapist and client as the work together to discuss the effect of the new behavior or belief. NCLT therapist understand that most clients, while stating that they desire improvement, really like and wish to hold on to their existing behaviors and beliefs. This is because they have worked hard to learn them and they are in many instances automatic. Leaving the resolution of conflict solely for the client to do increases the probability that the new information may be rejected. In addition, if it does get included the way that it gets included, may be neither what the therapist intended nor desirable. The therapist should of course be aware that in some instances, where beliefs are rigidly held, it is easier for an individual to reject the new information to preserve the core belief.

New Information Is Appended onto Existing Information

New information is not learned snippet by snippet and retained in isolation. New information is appended onto existing information. This implies that you cannot just add an adaptive response or thought onto what is an already existing body of maladaptive behaviors and thoughts. NCLT recognizes that entire clusters of thoughts related to certain topic and actions will have to be critically challenged and altered. We will have more to say about this topic a little later.

2. **There is no knowledge independent of the meaning attributed to it by prior experience. Knowledge is constructed by the client.**

This principle relates to principle number one in that no information is processed by an individual independently of what that individual already knows. As we have seen, this principle is directly related to the known functioning of working memory. New information is always appended to existing memory in order to be remembered. This principle is also entirely consistent with constructivist learning models.

According to Piaget there are no pure facts if by "facts are meant phenomena presented nakedly to the mind by nature itself, independently respectively of the hypothesis by means of which the mind examines them and of the systematic framework of existing judgments into which the observer pigeon-holes every new observation" (Piaget, 1974, p. 33).

This principle has a number of implications, but especially highlights how the therapist would benefit by understanding how new information is likely to be received by the individual. If the therapist is going to provide information designed to alter a maladaptive belief or set of beliefs (depression), it is necessary to identify for both the therapist and the client how that existing set of beliefs operate and how they distort new information to conform to existing thought patterns. For example, how is talking about children, even in a manner deemed healthy by the therapist, going to be interpreted in the mind of another parent versus that of a childless adult? How is talking about the fine meal you had in the steak restaurant last night going to be interpreted in the mind of a vegetarian?

As can readily be seen, there are a multitude of discussions that occur in any therapeutic encounter of any sort that provide hypothetically neutral information that may be interpreted by the client in any number of adaptive or maladaptive ways. Making these associations explicit and discussable is an essential task of therapy. The client or therapist who does not understand this principle operates at considerable peril. The examination of how the existing schema encodes information should be the primary task of the intervention and should occur before the actual attempts at altering are made. Without this information it is possible, and in some instances likely, that those maladaptive beliefs and behaviors will actually be reinforced by the therapeutic intervention.

3. **In therapy it is the client who decides which sensory input is important, to construct meaning out of and commit to memory.**

Clients in therapy do not consider everything said during the course of therapy as important or worthy of retention in memory. This selective attention is not unique to therapy. Studies suggest that as much as 30% of the material provided during a lecture is already lost by the conclusion of the lecture (Prince, 2004). Listeners actively choose which information to attend to and remember. Changing what clients attend to is more important that what clients actually practice telling themselves (Greenberg & Safran, 1981). This process of selected attention to specific material, and the ignoring of other material, is termed gating. We will talk more about gating later.

What is important to remember now is that clients, not therapists, ultimately get to determine what is important and what it not, and it is highly possible that clients may select things to attend to that are extraneous to the process of treatment. NCLT therapists understand this process and engage actively with their clients to help them focus on critical areas of the materials to be learned.

4. **The construction of meaning in therapy is a purposeful activity.**

Clients learn to learn as they learn. This is because as they learn they construct systematically more advanced and complex adaptive schema (bodies of knowledge).

It is the construction of the schema that determines how new knowledge is both interpreted and potentially incorporated. Once learned, clients subconsciously rehearse and refine these new schemas and related strategies to move them towards automaticity (Thatch, 1997).

Automaticity

From the time we come into this world we are practicing learning. We are practicing the learning of new behaviors. The goal of practice is to reach a level of automaticity, or the ability to engage in these routines without having to apply our mental resources to the process (Wasserman & Wasserman, 2015). The intent is to free our mental resources to apply to new experiences. The effect is that through the process of learning these practiced elements become automatic. Motor behaviors, cognitions, and emotional states all follow the same principles of learning, and ultimately, those which are well practiced, or consistently experienced, become automatic. Most of these automatic elements are adaptive. Some are not.

At the beginning of therapy a client will present with a number of problem behaviors, emotional reactions, and/or ideas which are causing them distress. These behaviors, emotions, and ideas are the result of a complex and extensive learning history that, through the continuing interaction between existing schema and new information in the environment, produced the current automatic default condition.

Learning in therapy consists both of constructing meaning and constructing new systems of interrelated meaning. The goal of this learning is to develop a system of adaptive behavior and thought. In most instances this new system of adaptive behavior and thought will be at odds with the existing and entrenched system of maladaptive behavior and thought. In order to make therapeutic progress, the new system of adaptive behavior and thought must be reinforced and encouraged to the point of automaticity, while the existing maladaptive schema must be made nonautomatic. This is a two pronged process. The new adaptive system must be purposefully selected and practiced, while at the same time the old maladaptive system must be purposefully deselected and not practiced.

All of this requires precision in definition and in identifying therapeutic behavioral and emotional outcomes. It also requires that the client understand and participate in the process of constructing new and adaptive schema. Treatment will initially produce a new response schema that is poorly developed, skeletal, poorly generalized, and poorly interconnected. This mean that the client will likely not spontaneously use the new information outside of the therapeutic environment. This new schema must be purposefully developed and practiced to the point of automaticity. The client must be an active participant in this process. The process is best accomplished with clearly defined learning outcomes and specific teaching strategies designed to reach those outcomes. Individuals learn better and develop efficient subconscious rehearsal strategies when goals are clearly articulated (Dijksterhuis & Aarts, 2010). They cannot clearly articulate the outcome and processes unless those things are identified, and taught in the context of therapy.

Therapy therefore should be about the development or modification of schemas to produce a practiced, rich, and broadly generalized set of behaviors, emotions, and cognitions that are employed automatically when the situation requires.

5. **Humans learn by pattern matching. Each meaning we construct makes us better able to give meaning to other stimuli which can match with a previously identified and categorized, similar pattern.**

When we encounter a new stimuli, the brain immediately begins to attempt to match it with what is already known. Humans pattern match between crucial issues in the environment and elements of mental schemata to determine which schemata will be accessed and used to append the new information (Endsley & Garland, 2000). Classes of stimuli are grouped together in the brain.

Clients seeking treatment often have whole classes of stimuli (schemata) that they react poorly to. New stimuli are readily added, or appended to their existing schema. This is especially clear for clients with generalized anxiety disorders and depression. For example, imagine the client with a base of anxiety. They encounter a new situation, become anxious, the anxiety response becomes again, or consistently experienced. While this is largely true it is not always the case. On occasion, increasing exposure and information can amend a schemata or split it into two related schemata. Suppose, for example, you were afraid of all spiders and reacted with a great deal of anxiety to an appearance of any spider. Now suppose you were motivated by your new job at the arachnoid exhibit at the zoo and took the time to learn about spiders and found out which ones were dangerous and which were not. Eventually you would develop two highly related schemata, spiders which were dangerous and spiders which were not. The response patterns to these schemata would be different. Therapy should work in a similar fashion. The goal of treatment should be to make the response patterns of individual's to specific schema explicit so that they can be examined and modified. Maladaptive responses should be deconditioned, and adaptive responses practiced and automatized.

6. **The construction of meaning is neurophysiologically based and involves brain circuitry dedicated to pattern matching, learning, and reinforcement recognition.**

All information that is learned is processed over the same neural networks. There is no separate system for material learned in therapy, although there may be, as a result of the emotional valence of the material, different brain regions recruited for specific elements of what is discussed in treatment.

Specific recruitment of brain regions is not unique to learning in a therapeutic context it is a characteristic of all learning. Regions responsible for emotional valence and reward recognition are not the exclusive domain of the material learned in therapy. These regions are recruited by any activity which is accompanied by a level of arousal. The regions which are responsible for reward recognition are critical in the gating process. Gating is the process that determines what information is accepted into working memory and therefore determine what material is available to be worked on in therapy.

Therapists Knowingly or Unknowingly Provide Encouragement, Direction, and Support

Clearly the degree to which the relationship between the therapist and the client produces an environment for encouragement and support is a factor in determining the effect of therapy. It is clear that the therapists' approval and support is as source of reinforcement that is used by all therapists to guide and shape the course of learning.

7. **The language we use influences learning. Language and learning are inextricably intertwined.**

Language can impact and even restructure cognition (Diessel, 2014; Majid, Bowerman, Kits, Haun, & Levinson, 2004). The words we use and how we use them impact the way we feel and behave (Pennebaker & Francis, 1996). Research demonstrates that language use is a collaborative process that influences the representation of meaning in the speaker, the listener, and the collective that includes both the speaker and the listener (Holtgraves & Kahima, 2008). For therapy, this implies that both the client and the therapist would have meaning modified as a result of the language-based interaction. More importantly this implies that the therapists' participation is essential to the modification of meaning for the client. Finally, there is research that clearly identifies language as the scaffolding device unto which new thought is structured and developed (Clark, 2006).

What all of this implies is that language is a critical tool for the shaping and reshaping of thought and related emotional states. The directed, purposeful, and structured use of language is important for imparting information designed to change cognition. Obviously, the haphazard or inefficient use of this tool would produce less than optimal results. Therefore, those systems that make purposeful use of language are to be preferred to less directed systems where the expected impact of language is not planned, or in fact the use of language itself is minimized.

8. **Learning in therapy is a social activity. To be useful, knowledge acquired in therapy must be applied and practiced within the context of both new and existing relationships.**

There are two separate points here, the first of which is that learning is a social process with at least two active participants, and the second is that new learning must be practiced in those social contexts that it was intended to be used in. This practice must be purposeful and directed. The learning outcome for the practice should be known to the learner so that the result of the practice can be integrated into the appropriate body of existing knowledge. The goal is automaticity of new behavior into the repertoire of the individual.

A further point should be added in that learning without interaction between the person acting (the learner) and the social world as initially represented by the therapist is ineffective. To put it another way, it is not enough to just think about it, or talk about a new behavior or idea in the office. New behavior must be practiced in the social world for it to be incorporated into the automatic repertoire of the learner. Such practice represents the core of a planned and purposeful therapy process.

There is increasing recognition that cognition originates in basic motor movements and develops largely in social interaction shaped by cultural and environmental processes. These processes are central rather than incidental to cognitive development (Koziol & Budding, 2009; Watson-Gegeo, 2004).

The nature of the relationship between a therapist and a client can be conceptualized within this framework. The goal of the therapy is to provide a secure place in which new initial learning can take place that is free from threat and conducive to experimentation and practice. In this environment the therapist encourages, challenges, and then provides feedback on the progress of the learning.

9. **Learning in therapy is contextual. We learn in relationship to what else we already know, and what we already believe.**

People come into therapy with a history which is both experiential and knowledge based. In therapy it is not desirable to append adaptive knowledge to maladaptive pre-existing knowledge. To be effective, new skill sets and their associated cognitions must be developed and practiced. In practice this is difficult to do because humans show a strong tendency to hold onto prior knowledge and discount new knowledge that is not in agreement with prior knowledge. In other words, if the new knowledge disagrees with what I already know, I have a strong tendency to reject the new knowledge to protect my existing beliefs (Chinn & Brewer, 1993; Lipson, 1982). Indeed, it can be argued that one purpose of knowledge is to develop attitudes and belief systems that are resistant to change, and that this rejection of new knowledge serves a valuable protective function (Woods, Rhodes, & Biek, 1995).

In order to understand how this process works it is important to know that, as we have discussed, humans learn by pattern matching. When we first encounter a novel stimuli we search what we know, looking for similar patterns or constructs to relate it to (Carmicheal & Hayes, 2001). We then look at this information in light of what we already know. We can do of three basic things with this new knowledge. We can reject it and protect what we already know. We can consider it and see how it fits in with what we already know. Or we can accept it and alter what we already know. A prime example of this presented itself regarding people's belief as to whether or not the MMR vaccine caused autism. The symptoms of autism were often recognized at approximately the same time as the MMR vaccine was administered. Some people concluded that the vaccine was then the cause. This misinformation spread. Despite multiple attempts by the Center for Disease Control to debunk this myth, many held fast, and in some cases still do, to the cause and effect belief, rejecting the science to the contrary.

We must consider the psychological mindset with which people consider new information. New information can be perceived a "psychological threat." Cohen and Sherman (2014) suggest that people have a basic need to maintain the integrity of the self. Events that threaten self-integrity arouse stress and self-protective defenses that can hamper performance and growth. They point out that people may focus on the short-term goal of self-defense at the cost of long-term learning. Thus, psychological threat can impede adaptive change.

People tend to evaluate new information with a directional bias toward their existing belief set. New information has a number of properties among which is that it may be ambiguous, or it may be counter to existing belief sets. People tend to interpret ambiguous information in ways that are consistent with their existing views, or attitudinally congruent, and resist or outrightly reject information which is counter-attitudinal to their existing set (Lord, Ross, & Lepper, 1979; Taber & Lodge, 2006). In fact, research has demonstrated that the directional bias eclipses factual information. That is, presenting corrective information can not only fail to reduce misconceptions among resistant individuals, it can actually strengthen them (Nyhan & Reifler, 2010).

Steele (1988) first proposed the concept of self-affirmation which offers the explanation that people process in a manner which will protect their general self-integrity. This includes the need to protect their self from information which "threatens" their beliefs and attitudes by calling them into question. Steele found that individuals who felt secure in their self-worth did not engage in the process of dissonance reduction, that is, they were more open to new messages.

It is of importance to note, however, that having people engage in self-praise, or self-affirmations tends to backfire among low self-esteem individuals. This is believed to be because these "affirmations" lack credibility (Wood, Perunovic, & Lee, 2009). Therefore, the implication is that our clients who are most in need of improved self-esteem will least likely internalize a self-affirmation.

As we have seen, humans have a propensity to protect what we already know and therefore, the most likely scenario when confronted with new information is to outrightly reject it. The second most likely event is to consider it, and see how it fits in with what we already know. The least likely outcome is to readily accept the discordant new information and throw away, or irrevocably alter what we already know. Much of what the lay person thinks about when they think about therapy is defined by this last, most unlikely outcome. People believe that the therapist will say something, and on the basis of that statement, a transformation of the maladaptive body of knowledge will occur. As we have just learned, this is both unlikely and counter to the actual tendency of people when they encounter new information.

What is more likely, and in fact therapeutically desirable, is that the client (learner) engages in the middle option. They will use the new information to see how it relates to what they already know. We do know a few things about how this occurs. One of the most important things is that for this objective analysis to occur, the learner must be motivated to do the comparison, and dispassionate about the analysis. The stronger the attitude is held, the more difficult the comparison is to make (Woods et al., 1995). In addition, beliefs associated with strong affect states lead to strongly held attitudes which are more resistant to change.

All of this goes to the point that in order to change the strongly held, emotionally laden belief systems that characterize the thinking of people with emotional problems, the clients must be encouraged to do a systematic, and dispassionate analysis of those belief systems in an environment, or in a manner that does not threaten the client and cause the client to withdraw. Based on constructivist principles such as the "just right challenge" (Vygotsky, 1934/1986) new information must be just different enough and minimally threatening enough to enable the client to process it while at the same time be both novel and interesting enough to encourage the allocation of working memory. This calls for a careful and thoughtful assessment of the type of new information, its purpose, and how it will be offered to the client. This argues persuasively that clients should not be left to their own devices to filter the information provided in a therapeutic exchange because their natural tendency will be to reject new information or avoid comparison or questioning their passionately held attitudes. The job of the therapist is, with the learning outcome clearly in mind, to systematically prepare the stimuli so that they meet the just right challenge and create an environment wherein the client is open to and engaged in confronting maladaptive attitudes and beliefs. By a process of shaping and desensitization, the therapist should present new information designed to challenge the existing attitude, while at the same time not being threatening to it.

10. **It is not possible to assimilate new knowledge without having some structure developed from previous knowledge upon which to build.**

Learning is incremental. The more we know, the more we can learn. Therefore, any effort to teach must be connected to the state of the client, and must provide a clear, direct, and unambiguous path into the subject for the learner that emanates from the learner's (client's) previous knowledge. This implies that adaptive beliefs and constructs should form the basis of new learning, and that therapy should be directed towards both creating the functional beliefs, attitudes, and skills sets, and then practicing those skills sets in multiple environments.

There is research that clearly indicates that learning occurs when potential responses to internal representations of environmental occurrences are reweighted, with some responses being made more likely and other responses becoming less likely. This data suggests that older conceptions, once demonstrated to be incorrect, have their internal representations changed (Petrov, Dosher, & Lu, 2005). Change implies that the predictive weights of the response are reweighted, resulting in some responses being much more likely to occur than others. In other words, learning occurs when some responses are trained and selected, and others are not trained and are deselected. Learning is effective when this process is directed and specific, with the learning paths specified and reinforced. Learning is then enhanced through a process of refinement of, and automization of, these selected responses (Neches, 1987).

11. **Learning new ideas and ways of behaving in therapy is not instantaneous.**

Learning requires both practice and rewards. Learning theory identifies this as the Laws of Effect/Exercise (Thorndike, 1932). Meaningful and utilitarian learning requires the revisiting of ideas in many contrasts and situations. Clients must recognize old ideas as maladaptive, and actively seek to replace them with new ideas based upon a foundation of new learning and successful application. Research has suggested that learning new skills or changing existing cognitive schema is enhanced, in terms of increased automaticity, when new concepts are pulled into working memory and then used in multiple applications (Logan, 1992). In order to create these various applications, guided practice enhanced with behavioral practice improves learning efficiency (Felder & Brent, 2003) increasing the likelihood of the change being rewarding.

There is a delicate balance required when learning complex material in therapy. Research indicates that cognitive load-reducing methods are effective to reach high rates of retention of information and behavior for complex tasks. These cognitive load-reducing methods include low variability of presentation, complete guidance, and feedback. Once the new information is acquired, it is precisely these methods that hinder the transfer of learning to new situations. In order to effect generalization, methods that induce appropriate and increasing cognitive load, such as high variability and limited guidance or feedback, increase effective learning (van Merriënboer, Kester, & Paas, 2006). In other words, to effect learning and generalization of new constructs in therapy, initially, highly structured and guided instruction is necessary to create the new schema. Only after the new schema is constructed it is beneficial to reduce guidance and structure, which will then increase the cognitive demand on the client and thereby facilitate generalization and application of the new skill.

Is There an "Aha" Moment in Therapy?

People assume that during the course of treatment a therapist will say something and all of a sudden a magic moment of realization and awareness will occur. It will be sudden, and often occur in response to a single thing the therapist has said. This is referred to as the "Aha" moment. Is there then an "Aha" experience in neurocognitive learning therapy and if so what is the explanation for it?

The easiest answer is both yes and no. Yes, because after sufficient guided instruction, clients will develop a new way of looking at things and begin to change their behavior as a result of this newly modified cognitive schema. From the moment that the schema is reconceptualized (assimilation) new information will be filtered through it, and as a result will not be thought of, or reacted to, in the same way as it had been in the past. No, because the change does not come easily, or in fact suddenly. It is hard won, and the result of initially structured, and focused, guided practice and repetition.

Consider, for example, our well-practiced schema about our solar system and the planets in it. In 2006, however, astronomers announced that Pluto was no longer a planet because of its size and lack of domination of its orbital environment. It had been reclassified. We all went to bed one night safe in the notion that we knew Pluto was a planet, and woke up the next day to find out that it wasn't. It was an "Aha" moment to be sure, but it couldn't have occurred without us first knowing what a planet was and having a basic understanding of the solar system. It could not have arrived without the countless hours of investigation and scientific discussion that preceded the decision about what schema to include Pluto in. Much as Piaget and Vygotsky suggested, there came a moment when new information altered our schema of the solar system and planet Pluto. But, we needed to have a schema in the first place in order for it to be altered.

An example of a changed schema in clinical work would be one wherein a young woman believes that she has been a poor parent and the cause of her child being autistic. It is a historical truth that "refrigerator mothers" were once conceptualized as the etiological agent of autism (Demaria, Aune, & Jodlowski, 2008). The schema regarding the etiology of autism changed twice; Once when refrigerator mothers were included, and again when they were removed. Our young client has been living with this guilt for 6 years. Imagine her guilt and the ensuing effect on the self-esteem of a woman who believed that her foremost role was to be a good mother. Now imagine teaching her about the current understandings regarding autism, and its lack of attribution to parenting.

Therapy works the same way. Current maladaptive response tendencies are reflective of a maladaptive learned and developed schema of responses. In order to alter a maladaptive schema, learning, repetition, and practice of new ways of thinking and new constructs must occur. The moment of change in the schema appears sudden, but in reality, it is the result of all that practice. For those of you who are concerned about the fate of poor Pluto, there is good news. There is a movement to try to have it reinstated as a planet. We all might wake up one morning and have to have another "Aha" experience. In fact, as we were writing this book, a new planet was apparently discovered. Our schema was required to change yet again. As clinicians, imagine the process you have taken clients through in order to correct the residual schema of the parent blaming either themselves, or their partner for their child being on the autism spectrum. In all likelihood, the answer you provided regarding current beliefs of the etiology was questioned several times. As your client came to have a greater understanding of the multiple "causes" of autism, they experienced an "Aha" moment.

We are not alone conceptualizing the development of maladaptive cognitive response sets as modifying cognitive schema's in line with constructivist learning theory. Research on therapy process has begun to identify this course of schema change as part of therapy, and develop ways to assess it. For example, the assimilation model (Stiles, Meshot, Anderson, & Sloan, 1992) proposes and evaluates for a systematic sequence of changes in the representation of a problematic experience during psychotherapy. The model is supported by research that indicates increasing degrees of assimilation of insights as therapy progresses.

12. **Motivation is a key component in learning. Not only is it the case that motivation helps learning, it is essential for learning.**

Poorly motivated clients, especially in the world of adolescent therapy, are the bane of clinical practice. Parents complain about their poorly motivated children, and bring them to therapists to properly motivate them, perhaps particularly about school. Historically, therapy does a poor job of doing so. NCLT has its own take on motivation, and it is one that allows for effective intervention in this area of clinical practice.

For NCLT, motivation is not the product of a mystical personality trait that certain individuals either have in abundance, or in which they are deficit. For NCLT, motivation reflects the operation of the reward recognition circuit, which is either more or less efficiently integrated with behavioral circuits. A client may state, and are serious when doing so, that they are motivated to change, but in particular may be unmotivated to engage in the behaviors necessary to facilitate that learning. They desire the outcome, but the component behaviors are not rewarding and therefore not engaged. The key to addressing this situation therapeutically is to remember that success brings reinforcement, and the increased likelihood that the action will continue to be selected in the future. Therapeutic progress, therefore, is facilitated when a planned program of increasingly complex actions is engaged in and reinforced. Motivation is therefore derived from successful practice and automatization of target behaviors designed to achieve a specific goal.

Motivation, in the NCLT model, is defined as the contribution of the reward system to the allocation of working memory and stimulus selection for response. Motivation involves multiple brain systems operating in concert. In this regard, brain regions cannot be simply labeled as either contributing, or not contributing, to motivated behavior. Rather, it is necessary to consider the specific circumstances under which the region is being engaged (McGinty et al., 2011).

Reward Recognition and Motivation

"Reward is a central component for driving incentive-based learning, appropriate responses to stimuli, and the development of goal-directed behaviors. In order to understand the role reward recognition has for learning new things, it is important to understand how different brain regions are recruited to work together to evaluate environmental stimuli and transform that information into actions" (Haber & Knutson, 2010, p. 4). The operation and integration of these reward recognition circuits and their importance are discussed later on. As pertains to motivation, recent research clearly indicates that reinforcement plays a crucial role as to what is selected for attention and what is not. The reward recognition circuit is essential for gating (selecting) knowledge to be attended to, and subsequently learned (Wasserman & Wasserman, 2015). This is because what is gated, or attended to, is what is admitted to working memory, and also determines what is retrieved from long-term store by pattern recognition (Shell et al., 2010). What gets retrieved by pattern recognition depends on the reward history, idiosyncratic to the individual client. Therefore, motivation in this model is the strength of the reward history and current reward valuation of the external stimulus as it pertains to the reward history of the individual.

Reward Recognition Circuitry

Reinforcement valuation and appraisal can be looked at as the driver of the constellation of behaviors associated with motivation because it determines the recruitment of various neural network components for a particular task. It also serves to orient and behaviorally direct the individual to a particular subset of environmental stimuli. In support of this premise, Hart, Leung, and Balleine (2014) point out that "considerable evidence suggests that distinct neural processes mediate the acquisition and performance of goal-directed instrumental actions. Whereas a cortical-dorsomedial striatal circuit appears critical for the acquisition of goal-directed actions, a cortical-ventral striatal circuit appears to mediate instrumental performance, particularly the motivational control of performance" (p. 104). While they point out that these distinct circuits of learning and performance constitute two distinct "streams" controlling instrumental conditioning, the interface between these two streams or circuits might represent a juncture for a limbic-motor interface. They posit that the basolateral amygdala, which is heavily interconnected with both the dorsal and ventral subregions of the striatum, coordinates this interaction, providing input to the final common path to action. NCLT theory posits that this interface represents the intersection of the reward circuitry that creates and maintains motivation and engagement (Wasserman & Wasserman, 2015).

13. **Maladaptive behavior and thought based upon automaticity.**

Given the limited capacity of working memory, automaticity is the goal of human learning (Aarts & Dijksterhuis, 2000; Bargh & Chartrand, 1999). In this regard, maladaptive thought and resulting behavior follow the same principles of automaticity. It is no different than any other type of thought, including adaptive thought. It is learned in the same way, automatized the same way, and expressed behaviorally in the same way. The neural circuitry involved in its learning is the same neural circuitry that is involved in all other learning. From this we can conclude that the neural circuitry itself, over which the maladaptive learning took place, is functioning appropriately. A corollary of this is that it is not guaranteed that a person with an emotional dysregulation issue has a badly wired brain. It is rather that the learned connections, or resulting neurophysiologically strengthened connectivity, leads to less than adaptive behavior and thought. Imagine the child who was colic as an infant. They had difficulties regulating their physiological states. This difficulty represents a developmental inefficiency in the system, rather than a broken or badly wired system. Although the research suggests that more of these children will go on to develop anxiety-based disorders, not all of them do. If, however, this emotional dysregulation pattern persisted, it would eventually become highly practiced, rendering it neurophysiologically efficient, but behaviorally dysfunctional.

This leads to an interesting likelihood; That in many instances, including discussions regarding nosology or etiology, where behavioral definitions of mental health issues are utilized, brains are not defectively, permanently wired, or permanently damaged. In many instances, the diagnosis merely implies that the current patterns of connectivity are the result of reinforcement patterns that have not produced adaptive behavior. NCLT posits that, in most instances, this is not a permanent condition. These pathways supporting maladaptive behavior can be altered by the same processes that supported their formation in the first place.

14. **The ability to solve problems and the ability to adapt to novel situations are positively correlated with improved mental health.**

Learning occurs when potential responses to internal representations of environmental occurrences are reweighted with some responses being made more likely and other responses becoming less likely (Petrov et al., 2005). Both working memory and processing speed efficiency, which impacts the quality or quantity of information represented, play important roles in this process. Deselection and reselection depends on the ability to suppress (deselect) newly identified task-irrelevant information as well as the ability to activate (select) newly identified task-relevant information (Brewin & Beaton, 2002). Interestingly, increased working memory and processing speed efficiency are both associated with fluid intelligence, and are associated with the ability to suppress unwanted stimuli and impulses.

Efficient working memory results in material being held in working memory for a greater period of time and being increasingly available for modification. This leads to the potential for increased flexibility. Increased flexibility in turn implies increased ability to evaluate novel solutions and consider new responses. It also suggests increased ability to select a new response to make automatic.

All of this suggests that fluid intelligence would be intimately and positively correlated with mental health. There is in fact some evidence that this might be the case, at least in populations of older individuals (Perlmutter & Nyquist, 1990).

15. **Therapy is cognitively demanding.**

Changes in patterns of thought, emotions, or behaviors require attention, cognitive effort, and energy. Deselection and reselection of a new process to make automatic (the process of therapy) is at first a conscious, planned, and time and energy consuming process. This is because conscious processes are focused and convergent, and draw heavily on limited working memory resources (Bays & Husain, 2008; Dijksterhuis & Meurs, 2006). There is also data that suggests that performance degradation, in terms of efficiency and fluidity, can occur when too much attention is allocated to processes that usually run more automatically (Bielock, Jellison, Rydell, McConnell, & Carr, 2006). Taken together this means that change requires significant mental effort. It means that an individual, who is attempting to eliminate a maladaptive, automatized process such as a complex maladaptive behavioral response or thought, will struggle due to the required cognitive effort. It is also likely that they will become inefficient and ineffective as they shift from their maladaptive strategies to newer, potentially effective, but not yet automatic cognitive processes. For example, a person who historically had a "snappy" comeback when they perceived themselves to be maligned may now not be able to generate a comment as they struggle to incorporate a new, assertive rather than aggressive style. They may perceive themselves as less competent than before. This moment in therapy will be highly discomforting to the patient, and the therapist must be prepared with strategies to continue to encourage the transition. Without planned and purposeful support, clients are likely to return to the previously automatized, but maladaptive processes.

16. **Learning is about connections in that what is stored together stays together in memory.**

Learning new things in therapy, as in all other learning, occurs in context. What is learned is associated and remembered in the context of what was around it during the time it was encountered. Therefore, it is critical to the process of therapy that newly learned, adaptive responses should be practiced in as many new contexts as possible. This practice should be a planned and purposeful part of treatment and not just left to circumstance.

The therapist should be highly cognizant of the fact that, given the right set of circumstances, inappropriate responses can be stored. Appropriate or socially acceptable responses can be stored with socially unacceptable responses should that association be reinforced. This is the basis for many fetishes and phobias. It is the basis for anxiety reactions (such as the student vomiting if there is a class test and carrying this behavior over to public speaking). Therapy should be designed to identify these maladaptive contextual pairings and where appropriate, work to repair appropriate emotional responses with acceptable behavioral outcomes.

These 16 principles reflect what is known from both learning theory and neuropsychological research. Whatever you call the result of the particular learning, self-actualization, behavioral change, spiritual growth, destruction of maladaptive gestalts, or behavior change, the result of therapy is that the individual engages in more adaptive behavior at the end than when they began. This inevitably means that the individual has learned new ways of behaving.

References

Aarts, H., & Dijksterhuis, A. (2000). Habits as knowledge structures: Automaticity in goal-directed behavior. *Journal of Personality and Social Psychology, 78*(1), 53–63. doi:10.1037/0022-3514.78.1.53.

Ablon, S., & Jones, E. (2002). Validity of controlled clinical trials of psychotherapy: Findings from the NIMH treatment of depression collaborative research program. *American Journal of Psychiatry, 159*(5), 775–783.

Bargh, J., & Chartrand, T. (1999). The unbearable automaticity of being. *American Psychologist, 54*(7), 462–479. doi:10.1037/0003-066X.54.7.462.

Bargh, J. A. (1992). The ecology of automaticity: Toward establishing the conditions needed to produce automatic processing effects. *American Journal of Psychology, 105*, 181–199.

Bays, P., & Husain, M. (2008). Dynamic shifts of limited working memory resources in human vision. *Science, 321*(5890), 851–854. doi:10.1126/science.1158023.

Bielock, S., Jellison, W., Rydell, R., McConnell, A., & Carr, T. (2006). On the causal mechanisms of stereotype threat: Can skills that don't rely heavily on working memory still be threatened? *Personality and Social Psychology Bulletin, 32*(8), 1059–1071. doi:10.1177/0146167206288489.

Brewin, C., & Beaton, A. (2002). Thought suppression, intelligence, and working memory capacity. *Behavior Research and Therapy, 40*(8), 923–930. doi:10.1016/S0005-7967(01)00127-9.

Chinn, C., & Brewer, W. (1993). The role of anomalous data in knowledge acquisition: A theoretical framework and implications for science instruction. *Review of Educational Research, 63*(1), 1–49. doi:10.3102/00346543063001001.

Clark, A. (2006). Language, embodiment, and the cognitive niche. *Cognitive Sciences, 10*(8), 370–374.

Cohen, G. L., & Sherman, D. K. (2014). The psychology of change: Self-affirmation and social psychological intervention. *Annual Review of Psychology, 65*, 333–371.

Demaria, S., Aune, J., & Jodlowski, D. (2008). Bruno Bettleheim, autism and the rhetoric of scientific authority. In M. Osteen (Ed.), *Autism and representation* (pp. 65–77). New York: Routledge.

Diessel, H. (2014). Demonstratives, frames of reference, and semantic universals of space. *Language and Linguistics Compass, 8*(3), 116–132.

Dijksterhuis, A., & Aarts, A. (2010). Goals, attention, and (un)consciousness. *Annual Review of Psychology, 61,* 467–490.

Dijksterhuis, A., & Meurs, S. (2006). Where creativity resides: The generative power of unconscious thought. *Consciousness and Cognition, 15*(1), 135–146. doi:10.1016/j.concog.2005.04.007.

Elman, J., Bates, E., Johnson, M., Kanniloff-Smith, A., Parisi, D., & Plunkett, K. (1996). *Rethinking innateness: A connectionist perspective on development.* Cambridge: MIT Press.

Endsley, M., & Garland, D. (2000). *Situation awareness analysis and measurement.* Mahwah, NJ: Erlbaum.

Felder, R., & Brent, R. (2003). Learning by doing. *Chemical Engineering Education, 37*(4), 282–283.

Greenberg, L., & Safran, J. (1981). Encoding and cognitive therapy: Changing what clients attend to. *Psychotherapy: Theory, Research and Practice, 18*(2), 163–169. doi:10.1037/h0086076.

Haber, S., & Knutson, B. (2010). The reward circuit: Linking primate anatomy and human imaging. *Neuropsychopharmacology, 35*(1), 4–26.

Hart, G., Leung, B. K., & Balleine, B. W. (2014). Dorsal and ventral streams: The distinct role of striatal sub-regions in the acquisition and performance of goal-directed actions. *Neurobiology of Learning and Memory, 108,* 104–118. doi:10.1016/j.nlm.2013.11.00.

Holtgraves, T., & Kahima, Y. (2008). Language, meaning, and social cognition. *Personality and Social Pyschology Review, 12*(1), 173–194. doi:10.1177/1088868307309605.

Klin, A., Shultz, S., & Jones, W. (2015). Social visual engagement in infants and toddlers with autism: Early developmental transitions and a model of pathogenesis. *Neuroscience and Biobehavioral Reviews, 50,* 189–203. doi:10.1016/j.neubiorev.2014.10.006.

Koziol, L. F., & Budding, D. E. (2009). *Subcortical structures and cognition: Implications for neuropsychological assessment.* New York: Springer.

Lipson, M. (1982). Learning new information from text: The role of prior knowledge and reading ability. *Journal of Literacy Research, 14*(3), 243–261. doi:10.1080/10862968209547453.

Logan, G. D. (1992). Attention and preattention in theories of automaticity. *American Journal of Psychology, 105,* 317–339.

Lord, C. G., Ross, L. R., & Lepper, M. R. (1979). Biased assimilation and attitude polarization: The effects of prior theories on subsequently considered evidence. *Journal of Personality and Social Psychology, 39*(11), 2098–2109.

Majid, A., Bowerman, M., Kits, S., Haun, D., & Levinson, S. (2004). Can language restructure cognition? The case for space. *Trends in Cognitive Neuroscience, 8*(3), 108–114. doi:10.1016/j.tics.2004.01.003.

McGinty, V., Hayden, B., Heilbronner, S., Dumont, E., Graves, S., Mirrione, M., et al. (2011). Emerging, reemerging, and forgotten brain areas of the reward circuit: Notes from the 2010 motivational and neural networks conference. *Behavioural Brain Research, 225,* 348–357. doi:10.1016/j.bbr.2011.07.036. Retrieved from National Institute of Health.

Neches, R. (1987). Learning through incremental reinforcement of procedures. In D. Klahr, P. Langley, & R. Neches (Eds.), *Production system models of learning and development* (pp. 163–222). Boston: Massachusetts Institute of Technology.

Nyhan, B., & Reifler, J. (2010). When corrections fail: The persistence of political misperceptions. *Political Behavior, 32*(2), 303–330.

Pennebaker, J., & Francis, M. (1996). Cognitive, emotional, and language processes in disclosure. *Cognition and Emotion, 10*(6), 601–612.

Perlmutter, M., & Nyquist, L. (1990). Relationship between self-reported physical and mental health and intelligence performance across adulthood. *Journal of Gerontology, 45,* 145–155.

Petrov, A., Dosher, B., & Lu, Z. (2005). The dynamics of perceptual learning: An incremental reweighting model. *Psychological Review, 112*(4), 715–743. doi:10.1037/0033-295X.112.4.715.

Piaget, J. (1972). Development and learning. In C. S. Lavattelly (Ed.), *Reading in child behavior and development.* New York: Harcourt Brace Janovich.

Piaget, J. (1974). *The child's conception of the world.* London: Paladin Books.

Piaget, J. (1977). *Intellectual evolution from adolescence to adulthood.* Cambridge: Cambridge University Press.

Regan, A., & Hill, C. (1992). Investigation of what clients and counselors do not say in brief therapy. *Journal of Counseling Psychology, 39*(2), 168–174. doi:10.1037/0022-0167.39.2.168.

Rutter, M. (2006). *Genes and behavior: Nature-nurture interplay explained.* Malden, MA: Blackwell Publishing.

Shell, D., Brooks, D., Trainin, G., Wilson, K., Kauffman, D., & Herr, L. (2010). *The unified learning model how motivational, cognitive, and neurobiological sciences inform best teaching practices.* New York: Springer.

Steele, C. M. (1988). The psychology of self-affirmation: Sustaining the integrity of the self. In L. Berkowitz (Ed.), *Advances in experimental social psychology* (Vol. 21, pp. 261–302). New York: Academic Press.

Taber, C. S., & Lodge, M. (2006). Motivated skepticism in the evaluation of political beliefs. *American Journal of Political Science, 50*(3), 755–769.

Thatch, W. (1997). Context-response linkage. *International Review of Neurobiology, 41*, 599–611. doi:10.1016/S0074-7742(08)60372-4.

Thorndike, E. (1932). *The fundamentals of learning.* New York: Teachers College Press.

van Merriënboer, J., Kester, L., & Paas, F. (2006). Teaching complex rather than simple tasks: Balancing intrinsic and germane load to enhance transfer of learning. *Applied Cognitive Psychology, 20*(3), 343–352. doi:10.1002/acp.1250.

Vygotsky, L. (1934/1986). *Thought and language.* Cambridge: MIT Press.

Wampol, B. (2015). How important are the common factors in psychotherapy? An update. *World Psychiatry, 14*(3), 270–277. doi:10.1002/wps.20238.

Wasserman, T., & Wasserman, L. (2015). The misnomer of attention deficit hyperactivity disorder. *Applied Neuropsychology: Child, 4*(2), 115–122. doi:10.1080/21622965.2015.1005487.

Watson-Gegeo, K. (2004). Mind, language, and epistemology: Toward a language socialization paradigm for SLA. *Modern Language Journal, 88*(3), 331–350. doi:10.1111/j.0026-7902.2004.00233.x.

Wood, J. V., Perunovic, W. Q. E., & Lee, J. W. (2009). Positive self-statements; power for some peril for others. *Psychological Science, 20*(7), 860–866.

Chapter 2
The Theoretical Basis for Neurocognitive Learning Therapy

Neurocognitive learning therapy is based on contributions from three branches of science; learning theory, small world hub models of cognitive processing, and epigenetics. Before we proceed to further discuss the didactics of the model, it would be wise to spend some time discussing the foundation science upon which NCLT rests. This will serve two purposes. The first is to have the reader understand that there are solid and empirically valid reasons for the practice of NCLT. The second is more pragmatic. The second purpose is to enable the reader to understand the reasons for the choice of goals and learning objectives in therapy.

Learning Theory and NCLT

NCLT is heavily indebted to the unified learning model (ULM) (Shell et al., 2010), and also combines elements from constructivist, but especially connectionist cognitive learning models, neuropsychology, and basic learning theory.

What Is the Unified Learning Model?

The unified learning model (ULM) integrates three aspects of cognition: (a) crystallized intelligence (knowledge) as represented by accumulated knowledge stored in long-term memory, (b) fluid intelligence as represented by working memory capacity, and (c) motivation, which is considered to be a driver of working memory allocation. Like the ULM, NCLT is based on a rather simple premise that these three components underlie all of human learning.

Working memory is defined as temporary storage and processing of information. Critical to the understanding of how NCLT operates is the idea that how working memory is constructed and operates, determines how things are learned. Working

© Springer International Publishing AG 2017
T. Wasserman, L.D. Wasserman, *Neurocognitive Learning Therapy: Theory and Practice*, DOI 10.1007/978-3-319-60849-5_2

memory stores information in identifiable patterns (schemas in constructivist models) that are retrieved from long-term store when new information is encountered. Working memory is based on prior knowledge, which is in turn based on the network's response to a novel stimuli it receives. Remember, motivation is the driving force behind working memory. Very simply, if I am motivated by something, I will be willing to allocate my working memory to attending to and learning it.

Knowledge

Knowledge essentially is defined as every piece of information we have stored within long-term memory. Knowledge has a twofold role. Remembering that the purpose of learning is to increase the data in long-term storage (increase or change knowledge), knowledge is what results from the proper functioning of working memory. Knowledge also reciprocally influences the functioning of working memory. That is because the way working memory encodes new information is directly constrained by the existing knowledge base in long-term memory. This is because new knowledge is constantly being compared to, and appended upon, old knowledge. New and old knowledge meet in memory store. The result of this meeting is that each works upon the other and produces new knowledge, which is then returned to long-term memory. This is important to understand for the therapeutic process, because knowing this accounts for the individuality and uniqueness of each person who creates knowledge. Because individual experiences vary, no two sets of knowledge stores are identical.

Motivation

While there are many definitions and models of motivation, the ULM and NCLT define motivation quite specifically as the impetus for directing working memory and attention, to a particular task. Motivation is therefore, along with attention, an essential component of working memory.

The interplay of the components results in the three basic principles of learning for the ULM, and for NCLT, which have their implications for therapeutic learning. They are:

1. Learning is a product of working memory allocation
2. Working memory's capacity for allocation is affected by prior knowledge
3. Working memory allocation is directed by motivation

In clinical practice terms, people only learn what they pay attention to, and what they pay attention to is directed by what they already know and what they find reinforcing. Clinically speaking, this means that if I determine that the pattern match of a new incoming stimulus is reinforcing, I will allocate my working memory to it and learn it. It also means, however, that if I perceive the new stimuli to pattern match as a threat then I will feel anxious and threatened.

General Rules of Learning in NCLT

NCLT has principles of learning that are based upon the neurobiology of learning and are incorporated into the therapeutic interaction for a vertical brain model. These are as follows:

1. New learning requires attention. Only those items that are being attended to will be candidates for working memory store.
2. Learning is pattern recognition. Those patterns that are recognized and routinely retrieved from store are utilized and generalized. We would add that those patterns are also associated by repetition and reinforcement to the arousal centers located in the limbic system. When retrieved from memory store, they are accompanied by their associated emotional response set. Any new learning is attached to existing schemas, and each set of these existing schemas has a motivational and emotional response associated with it.
3. Learning is about connection. What is learned together is stored together in memory. What is stored together stays together in memory. Appropriate or socially acceptable responses can be stored with socially unacceptable responses should that association be reinforced. Given the right set of motivational circumstances, inappropriate responses can be stored.
4. The goal of learning is automaticity. That is, the goal of learning is to have complex connections between elements of data available to the learner without effort. Clinically speaking, that means that once a response pattern is automatized, people will automatically associate and continue to associate emotional states with events, without cognitive effort to change those associations. One goal of therapy is to make new, essential connections as efficient and automatic as possible. This is because active working memory and transfer of information involves effort, and the amount of effort that people can expend is physiologically limited (Callicott et al., 1999).

    A procedure that has achieved automaticity can run itself. When these automatic response chains produce maladaptive procedures, and we must change an automated process, we must de-automatize it. This is the process of therapy. Our model recognizes that to de-automatize a maladaptive procedure, and create a new adaptive procedure, specific, directed allocation of attentional resources is required. This concept is important as it implies a more directed and targeted process than what is used in many nondirective approaches. Without directed allocation of working memory, nondirective approaches result in many false starts, and allocation of working memory to procedures that would not, in the end, result in adaptation.

5. Learning requires repetition. Automaticity is achieved through practice and generalization.
6. Learning is learning. While all neurons learn in exactly the same way, people utilize these processes idiosyncratically.
7. Motivation is particular to the individual.

Learning is the product of a consistent and ongoing interaction between the individual's experiences and their genetically derived predispositions. This interaction has been termed epigenetics (Elman, 1993). Epigenetics basically posits that behaviors and experiences interact with physiological, cognitive, and emotional predispositions to produce current behavior (Atzaba-Poria, Pike, & Deater-Deckard, 2004; Buehler & Gerard, 2013). Available research suggests that current behavior reflects the accumulation of all these interactive events. Rutter (2006) points out that a number of factors including susceptibility genes, environmentally mediated causal risk processes, nature-nurture interplay, the effects of psychosocial adversity on the organism, the causal processes responsible for group differences in rates of disorder, and age-related changes in psychopathological characteristics all play a part in the development of complex adaptive and maladaptive behavior.

The Goal of Therapy Is Also Competence

The term competence has been used to refer to accumulated learning experiences that result in a pattern of effective adaptation within an environment. Within the NCLT clinical context, it implies that the individual has (or lacking competence does not have) the capability to perform well in the future. Like many cognitive therapy models, NCLT posits that an individual who lacks competence in an environment becomes self-aware and engages in negative self-appraisals. These negative self-appraisals are reinforced and reproduced regularly, until they are automatically associated with a class of behaviors or physiological responses. NCLT theory hypothesizes that these automatically associated physiological responses and appraisals are experienced as affect states such as depression and anxiety. That is, in part, because the physiological responses associated with these affect states are also associated, through the same principles of learning, to the cognitions associated with the appraisals. For example, imagine your client who, when in high school, on the debate team, came down with the flu and did very poorly when they had to engage in public speaking. They felt shaky, and it was hard for them to focus. These same feelings of "shakiness" and diminished focus occurred at the next debate. The student concluded that they are very anxious when they have to speak in public and tend to panic. This led to a concept of reduced competence secondary to negative self-appraisals. Through the process of therapy, the goal is to alter the competence of the client, and the self-perception of competence of the client. This in turn alters the client's physiological responses and eliminates, or reduces, maladaptive emotional associations and self-critical appraisals.

Specific learning experiences govern the development of the neural architecture to be sure, but the system's properties and functioning are governed by a constant and unchanging set of operational rules. Research has identified numerous neural structures that are involved in this network (McClure, York, & Montague, 2004). Essentially, this network governs reward processing and reward-dependent learning. McClure et al. (2004) identified a set of reward-related brain structures linked together in a small world connectionist system including the orbitofrontal cortex, amygdala, ventral striatum, and medial prefrontal cortex. Environmental experiences are evaluated in terms of their reward potential, and it is this determination that is the basis of what is learned and what isn't.

Knowledge Acquisition and Working Memory in Therapy

We can summarize what is learned in therapy. All of what is learned knowledge. NCLT offers the following as rules that govern the process of knowledge acquisition in therapy.

1. If knowledge in long-term memory is retrieved, the strength of association between all items retrieved to working memory is increased. Clinically, it must be remembered that how things are presented and grouped in working memory determines what procedures will be developed from their association.
2. If a knowledge is retrieved, all other elements of knowledge to which it is connected are retrieved, and all connections are strengthened.
3. If parts of retrieved knowledge match to working memory contents, the connection between the existing knowledge and the new material are strengthened. If parts of retrieved knowledge do not match to contents in working memory, the connections are weakened and inhibited. Establishing new pattern matches (schemata) is an essential component in therapy.
4. If an action is successful, its connection to the knowledge of the situation in which it occurred is strengthened. If an action is unsuccessful, its connection to the knowledge of the situation in which it occurred is weakened or inhibited. The therapeutic implication of this is that new procedures must be understood and conscientiously practiced.
5. If knowledge has been retrieved, new information in working memory will be connected to this knowledge. This is the basis of establishing new adaptive procedures.
6. Any active knowledge in long-term memory is accessible to working memory.

Core Flexible Networks

Nomi et al. (2017) found that the human brain continually cycles through patterns of neural connections. They found that, most of the time, neural connections are agile, which they describe as fluid and flexible enough to meet presented challenges or mental tasks. In NCLT one major goal of therapy is to capitalize on core flexible neural networks that can be readily adapted to newly encountered situations. The core flexible networks (schemata) are the building blocks of the complex networks (routines) that will constitute the basis of our response to the ever changing demands presenting in the environment. Our model postulates that these practiced and thereby created complex network associations can be targeted and efficiently altered through direct instruction, thereby correcting prior maladaptive network recruitment patterns. That is not the entire goal of learning. What is also critical is that we assist in the production of a response tendency in the individual that would encourage that person to bring these networks to bear on new situations. That is, we must assist our client in getting to a state of readiness to bring the newly created network adaptations online more fluidly. There is increasing evidence of the regulatory control of these core flexible networks in the regulation of emotion and the development of mental dysfunction. For example, recent research points to the existence of a frontoparietal control system consisting of flexible hubs that regulate distributed systems of response according to task specific goals. Alterations of this control system have been identified in a wide range of mental diseases (Cole, Reposv, & Anticivic, 2014). Cole et al. (2014) suggested these flexible hubs reflect a critical role for the control system in promoting and maintaining mental health in that it implements feedback control to regulate symptoms as they arise, and when functioning correctly the system is protective against a variety of mental illnesses. The mission statement of therapy then is to target and promote the adaptive use of these control systems.

The Connectome and NCLT

The connectome is a term used to describe a comprehensive map of the neural white matter, or subcortical connections in the brain. The connectome is sort of a wiring diagram of the white matter connections between and amongst structures in an individual's brain. It is important to note that these connections are not hard wired. There are pathways and routes that are travelled, which are interlinked at neurochemical intersections, called synapses. These neurochemical interchanges allow sections of the pathway to be used for different routes connecting and reconnecting depending on task demands in the system for a response. This set up permits the same structure to be recruited for differing activities depending on the requirements of the task at hand and its perceived reward value.

A human brain is an amazingly complex organ containing some 700 trillion synaptic connections (*What Is the Connectome*, 2014). The synaptome is the term for the set of synaptic connections in a brain region. Each individual synapse is in itself highly complex, and acts as an independent switch to transmit cellular information. The synaptome is believed to be the site of learning, memory, and retrieval occurring at molecular states at each synapse of the connectome.

Any discussion of the connectome includes a discussion of a second type of brain matter, grey matter, which are the regions connected in the system by the white matter. Grey matter contains the cell bodies and axon terminals of neurons. It is where all synapses are located. The white matter, made up of axons, connects various grey matter areas (the locations of nerve cell bodies) of the brain to each other, and carries nerve impulses between neurons.

Understanding how white matter contributes to the information processing capabilities of the human brain has taken on increasing importance in the last 10 years as it is now recognized that it actively affects how the brain learns and functions. While grey matter is primarily associated with processing and cognition, white matter modulates the distribution of action potentials, acting as a relay and coordinating communication between different brain regions. White matter tracts are the structural highways of our brain, enabling information to travel quickly from one brain region to another region (van den Heuvel, Mandl, & Hulshoff-Pol, 2009).

The development of the connections of the human connectome is in large part, but not absolutely, due to the experiences that connectome has with the environment. As a result, the connectome is being continually shaped, formed, and altered by learning.

The Development of the Connectome and Psychopathology

The human connectome is the result of a complex developmental trajectory that insures the development of key neural networks that govern all aspects of cognition (Menon, 2013). Aberrations in the development of any of the networks contribute to psychopathology.

Humans are born with a functional but rudimentary connectome, organized in a stable, small world fashion, which integrates key networks to insure initial survival and support for future learning. Research also demonstrates heterogeneous pattern of changes across developing functional systems that map the external world onto the brain's attentional, sensory, emotional, and motivational subsystems (Menon, 2013).

NCLT recognizes that both environmental interaction and experience play a role in the development of the networks. The result of this interplay can lead to adaptive outcomes in learning and skills development, or to poor outcomes that are labeled as psychopathology.

Small World Hubs

One way to represent these networks is called graphical analysis. Graphical analysis is basically a statistically driven graph of the relationship between variables, in this case, brain regions. Bullmore and Sporns (2009) suggest that complex cognitive functioning is best represented by a connectionist small world hub model of neural networks. Small world neural network models are based on the concept of nodes which represent the confluence or connectivity points of neurons. Research has demonstrated that brain networks have characteristically small-world properties of dense or clustered local connectivity (nodes) with relatively few long-range connections to other similarly dense nodes. Nodes cluster together in small networks and vary to the degree of how central they are to the connections to other small clustered networks within the system. The nodes of a small world network have greater local interconnectivity or "cliquishness" than a random network, but the minimum path length between any pair of nodes is smaller than would be expected in a regular network.

Small-world networks are valuable models to use when evaluating the connectivity of nervous systems because the combination of high clustering and short path length between nodes provides a capability for the network to perform both specialized and modular processing in local neighborhoods and distributed or integrated processing over the entire network (Achard, Salvador, Witcher, Suckling, & Bullmore, 2006).

Is There Evidence that the Connectome Organizes Itself in Response to Learning?

A central premise of the NCLT model is that therapeutic learning impacts the organization of operation of the connectome and that the purpose of this reorganization is effective adaptation and the automatization of the more adaptive response. There is emerging research support that indicates that this premise is correct (Bar & DeSouza, 2016).

Brain imaging using magnetic resonance imaging (MRI) has revealed structural changes in white matter after learning complex tasks or behaviors. This line of research appears to indicate that white matter responds to experience in a manner that affects neuron function under normal circumstances, thereby affecting information processing and performance (Fields, 2010). There is evidence that white matter, especially myelin formation occurs during cognition, learning, development of skills, and memory. For example myelination of brain regions coincides with the development of specific academic and cognitive functions such as reading, development of vocabulary, and proficiency in executive decision making (Fields, 2008). These last two classes of skills are clearly associated with what happens in therapy. According to Fields (2010) when new skills are learned, the amount of myelin insulating an axon increases improving the ability of that neuron to signal. This leads to more efficient learning including reading, creating memories, playing a musical instrument, and more. A thicker sheath is also linked with better decision making. The purpose of learning is to improve efficiency, thereby encouraging automaticity.

Algorithms, Practice, Automatization, and NCLT

What then is automaticity in a learning theory context, and how might it be used in therapy? An automatic process is one that once initiated (regardless of whether it was initiated intentionally or unintentionally), runs to completion with no requirement for conscious guidance or monitoring (Moors & De Houwer, 2006). NCLT posits that the initiation of all automatic processes are conditional: They are all dependent on preconditions (e.g., the presence of a triggering stimulus, awareness of the stimulus, the intention that the process take place, a certain amount of attentional resources, and the salience of the stimulus). Automatic processes will vary with regard as to the specific subset of preconditions they require. The identification of these preconditions becomes an important element of the therapeutic process (Wasserman & Wasserman, 2016).

We will discuss automaticity in detail in a separate chapter, but the important thing here is that NCLT regards automatization as the goal of all learning, including the learning that occurs in therapy. This process can be represented by algorithmic models which attempt to represent brain functioning. An algorithm is a procedure or formula for solving a problem, which is based on conducting a sequence of specified actions depending upon the task it is being asked to do. A specific algorithm is a representation of a mathematically understandable and expressible specific cognitive process. These algorithmic models then represent processes as occurring in a small world hub model of brain organization. These algorithmic models support the idea that one learning mechanism accounts for the automatization of all complex cognitive routines. Algorithms have characteristics, one of which is the efficiency with which they run a particular process. The central theme of algorithm efficiency theories is that practice improves the efficiency (speed and fluidity) of the underlying algorithmic processes (Rawson, 2010). Consistent practice is therefore essential for the development of automaticity. Improvement in terms of efficiency requires algorithms to remain consistent with practice, even though aspects of the data they are practiced upon may change (Carlson & Lundy, 1992).

This principle holds in the clinical world as well, and would suggest that sound therapeutic process would involve systematic and direct practice of the new skill, which includes the complex combination of belief, emotion, and behavior, with the goal being automaticity. That is, the automatic, or the fluid and efficient ability to effortlessly utilize these new complex skills as needed. As stated, development of automaticity, or the development of the complex skill set, requires practice. This practice should include behaviors that devolve from the expression of the belief.

Change does not come from merely acknowledging some principle or idea. For example, it is not sufficient to merely agree with the statement that some charity is worthwhile. If a person develops an interest in a particular cause or charity, and begins to speak to others about its importance, as they "practice" this new skill, they will become more proficient at it. They will improve the speed at which they can recall points of view in their favor and become more efficient in their positional statements. Recalling these facts will consume less working memory effort as their speech becomes more automatic. This principle would also imply that the clearer the connection is between the belief and the practice, the more efficiently it will be learned.

The Implications of Algorithmic Models for Clinical Practice

There are additional features of algorithmic models that have implications for therapeutic practice. The algorithm (processing) strengthening (Adaptive Control of Thought or ACT) principle hypothesizes that the same algorithms responsible for the initial, nonautomatic stage of performance are also responsible for the skilled, automatic stage of performance. As practice continues, these algorithms are executed faster and more efficiently with increasingly less conscious allocation of working memory and control required. Automatic and nonautomatic algorithms differ only with regard to the features (such as speed and efficiency) they possess (Rawson, 2010).

Understanding, conceptually, how these algorithms operate is a helpful analogy for the therapist when designating intervention strategies because it mirrors the process which occurs across the connectome. It highlights that with practice, a set of routines will become the controlling sequence of the behavior, originating during the acquisition stage and maintained during the demonstration stage. Even for those of us who are "challenged by technology," we have all come to be familiar with internet searches. These searches are designed to go through a process and produce results. These processes are based on algorithms. An algorithm is a step by step procedure designed to solve a problem. The more a particular phrase is searched, the more frequently an algorithm is set into motion, increasing its speed and efficiency. This mirrors psychological cognitive, behavioral, and emotional patterns. That is, the establishment of the algorithm or cognitive/behavioral/emotional pattern will become, with practice, more automatic. The goal of therapy then is to make the healthy routine a stronger one which can be executed more easily and flexibly, ultimately becoming automatic.

Therapy Process in General NCLT in Specific

Most forms of therapy processes try to help clients identify triggers. NCLT is specific, emphasize identifying environmental triggers and altering the automatized response to them. Different therapy approaches vary on what the triggers they might focus on, how to identify them, and how to reprogram them, but all are in agreement that the task is the same; the reprogramming of maladaptive automatized responses into adaptive ones. Returning to our algorithms for a moment, the algorithm will initiate when presented with a trigger, in the case of the algorithm that may be a search phrase. Remember, the integrity of the search is only as "healthy" as the information initially presented. And the process will become faster and more efficient no matter what the trigger is. Therefore, therapy must be designed to help identify the trigger and reprogram the process.

The therapeutic questions to be derived from this observation are apparent and are specifically addressed by NCLT. Is there more than one efficient way to obtain this desired goal? If there are several ways to achieve this end, is one more efficient than the others? Is efficiency the goal, or is one process better at producing greater knowledge acquisition at the expense of time? Finally is there a particular form of therapeutic information provision that provides information in a manner that is consistent with how the brain is going to process it? These are all questions that deserve answers based on scientific inquiry and answers that NCLT attempted to provide.

NCLT emphasizes that automatized maladaptive behavioral and cognitive responses first be made available for working memory and attention, and systematically altered with the resulting adaptive behavior re-automatized. Identifying the triggers (preconditions) is an essential part of this process. For the most part, the maladaptive responses and the reformulated adaptive ones are learned. They do not "come preprogrammed at the factory." They represent the interaction of core temperamental characteristics (Chess & Thomas, 1967) and regulatory efficiency with environmental experiences.

Based upon small world hub models and the fact that individualized environmental experiences contribute to the development of the connectome NCLT posits that the network of connectionist hubs is unique to each human being. Some may be adaptive and some maladaptive, but the vast majority of these networks are developed based on the systems responses to the environmental stimuli it encounters. They are created by learning and are the result of that learning. In recognizing that, NCLT stresses that learning and educational processes and principles should be utilized when trying to alter them.

NCLT and Epigenetics

Recent research has made it increasingly clear that learning is based on changes in synaptic connections, and these changes in synaptic connections are effected by the products of specific genes which are expressed under specific conditions. Learning, therefore, is the product of a consistent and ongoing interaction between the individual's experiences and their genetically derived predispositions. This interaction has been termed epigenetics (Elman, 1993). Epigenetics basically posits that behaviors and experience interact with physiological, cognitive, and emotional predispositions to produce current behavior (Atzaba-Poria et al., 2004; Buehler & Gerard, 2013). Available research suggests that current behavior reflects the accumulation of all these interactive events. NCLT practice recognizes and discusses the role of epigenetics in the development and maintenance of mental health issues. NCLT recognizes that maladaptive response networks can also develop as a result of epigenetic and learning-based changes to the connectome. In these dysfunctional networks there would be no detectable structural abnormality or lesion, but rather differing patterns of connectivity leading to inefficient processing of information (Schmithorst, Wilke, Dardzinski, & Holland, 2005) or differing patterns of network activation (Thiel et al., 2014).

References

Achard, S., Salvador, R., Witcher, B., Suckling, J., & Bullmore, E. (2006). A resilient, low-frequency, small-world human brain functional network with highly connected association cortical hubs. *Journal of Neuroscience, 26*(1), 63–72. doi:10.1523/JNEUROSCI.3874-05.

Atzaba-Poria, N., Pike, A., & Deater-Deckard, K. (2004). Do risk factors for problem behaviour act in a cumulative manner? An examination of ethnic minority and majority children through an ecological perspective. *Journal of Child Psychology and Psychiatry, 45*(4), 707–718. doi:10.1111/j.1469-7610.2004.00265.x.

Bar, R., & DeSouza, J. (2016). Tracking plasticity: effects of long term rehearsal in expert dancers encoding music to movement. *PloS One, 11*(1), e147732. doi:10.1371/journal.pone.0147731.

Buehler, C., & Gerard, G. (2013). Cumulative family risk predicts increases in adjustment difficulties across early adolescence. *Journal of Youth and Adolescence, 42*(6), 905–920.

Bullmore, E., & Sporns, O. (2009). Complex brain networks: Graph theoretical analysis of structural and functional systems. National Review of Neuroscience, 10(3), 186–198. doi:10.1038/nrn2575.

Callicott, J., Mattay, V., Bertolino, A., Finn, A., Coppola, R., Frank, J., et al. (1999). Physiological characteristics of capacity constraints in working memory as revealed by functional MRI. *Cerebral Cortex, 9*(1), 20–26.

Carlson, R. A., & Lundy, D. H. (1992). Consistency and restructuring in cognitive procedural sequences. *Journal of Experimental Psychology: Learning, Memory, and Cognition, 18*, 127–141.

Chess, S., & Thomas, A. B. (1967). Behavior problems revisited: Findings of an anterospective study. *Journal of the American Academy of Child Psychiatry, 6*(2), 321–331.

Cole, M., Reposv, G., & Anticivic, A. (2014). The frontoparietal control system: A central role in mental health. Neuroscientist, 20(6), 652–664. doi:10.1177/1073858414525995.

Elman, J. (1993). Learning and development in neural networks: The importance of starting small. *Cognition, 48*(1), 71–99.

Fields, D. (2008). White matter in learning, cognition and psychiatric disorders. *Trends in Neuroscience, 31*(7), 361–370. doi:10.1016/j.tins.2008.04.001.

Fields, D. (2010). Change in the Brain's white matter the role of the brain's white matter in active learning and memory may be underestimated. *Science, 330*, 768–769. doi:10.1126/science.1199139.

McClure, S., York, M., & Montague, P. (2004). The neural substrates of reward processing in humans: The modern role of fMRI. *The Neuroscientist, 10*(3), 260–268. doi:10.1177/1073858404263526.

Menon, V. (2013). Developmental pathways to functional brain networks: Emerging principles. *Trends in Cognitive Science, 17*, 627–640. doi:10.1016/j.tics.2013.09.015.

Moors, A., & De Houwer, J. (2006). Automaticity: A theoretical and conceptual analysis. *Psychological Bulletin, 132*(2), 297–326. doi:10.1037/0033-2909.132.2.297.

Nomi, J. S., Vij, S. G., Dajani, D. R., Steimke, R., Damaraju, E., Rachakonda, S., et al. (2017). Chronnectomic patterns and neural flexibility underlie executive function. *Neuroimage, 147*, 861–871.

Rawson, K. (2010). Defining and investigating automaticity in reading. In B. Ross (Ed.), *The psychology of learning and motivation* (pp. 185–230). Burlington, NJ: Elsevier.

Rutter, M. (2006). *Genes and behavior: Nature-nurture interplay explained.* Malden, MA: Blackwell Publishing.

Schmithorst, V., Wilke, M., Dardzinski, B., & Holland, S. (2005). Cognitive functions correlate with white matter architecture in a normal pediatric population: A diffusion tensor MR imaging study. *Human Brain Mapping, 26*(2), 139–147.

Shell, D., Brooks, D., Trainin, G., Wilson, K., Kauffman, D., & Herr, L. (2010). *The unified learning model.* New York: Springer.

Thiel, A., Thiel, J., Oddo, S., Langnickel, R., Brand, M. M., & Stirn, A. (2014). CD-patients with washing symptoms show a specific brain network when confronted with aggressive, sexual and disgusting stimuli. *Neuropsychoanalysis*. doi:10.1080/15294145.2014.976649. Retrieved from http://www.tandfonline.com/doi/abs/10.1080/15294145.2014.976649#.VHVnSMlRaU9.

van den Heuvel, M., Mandl, R., & Hulshoff-Pol, H. (2009). Functionally linked resting-state networks reflect the underlying structural connectivity architecture of the human brain. *Human Brain Mapping, 30*(10), 3127–3141. doi:10.1002/hbm.20737.

Wasserman, T., & Wasserman, L. (2016). *Depathologizing psychopathology.* New York: Springer.

What is the connectome. (2014). Retrieved from The Brain Preservation Foundation: http://www.brainpreservation.org/content/connectome

Chapter 3
Eclecticism Redefined

Eclecticism, in a therapeutic context, is an approach to treatment that does not hold rigidly to a single model of unified treatment or set of assumptions concerning the etiology of disorders of mental health. The approach also does not specify a singular therapeutic intervention model, but instead relies on multiple components, each selected to address a particular presenting problem. An eclectic approach relies upon multiple theories, styles, or ideas to gain understanding of a subject, or applies different theories in particular cases to achieve specific outcomes. In sum, those therapists who practice eclecticism are not bound by the methodology, theories, or conventions of any one specific model. Instead, they may use what they believe or feel experience tells them will work best, either in general, or suiting the often immediate needs of individual clients, and working within their own preferences and capabilities as practitioners.

Most therapists acknowledge that they are functionally eclectic in treatment. That is because they adopt a number of differing therapeutic techniques to target the problems they encounter in treatment. Many of these techniques are quite successful in addressing the problems they are selected to address. The problem is that they do not hang together as an integrated whole. The problems they address are considered components, almost independent of each other. For example, relaxation exercises are often selected to address issues of anxiety, and correctly so, but without a model explaining the etiology of the anxiety, its maintenance, and how the anxiety might be related to other features of the clinical presentation. Or take for example the act of smiling. Smiling has been morphed into something now called smiling therapy. NCLT would posit that smiling clearly has therapeutic benefits. It is, however, a technique, not a therapy.

This state of affairs has been brought about due to the fact that there is not a unifying model of mental health that permits incorporating the various interventions into a logical and scientifically coherent integrated framework. This chapter will specify the ways in which NCLT integrates all treatment techniques into a coherent integrated model of mental health and its treatment.

© Springer International Publishing AG 2017

T. Wasserman, L.D. Wasserman, *Neurocognitive Learning Therapy: Theory and Practice*, DOI 10.1007/978-3-319-60849-5_3

Why Eclecticism

The core argument for eclectic approaches is that the therapist, instead of insisting upon strict adherence to one particular approach or school of thought, employs elements from a range of therapeutic techniques, with the goal of establishing a course that is personally tailored to the patient or client. The approach incorporates a variety of therapeutic principles and philosophies in order to create the ideal treatment program to meet the specific needs of the patient or client. Its adherents believe that it's a pragmatic approach to therapy based upon individualism and the uniqueness of each individual client (Grohol, 2015). The argument for this reasoning is that single model therapeutic approaches such as cognitive-behavior therapy or psychoanalysis unnecessarily "Pidgeon-hole" individuals and limit the effectiveness of treatment.

There are several systems of eclecticism. For example, technical eclecticism is designed "to improve the selection of the best treatment package for the client based on data on what has worked best for others in the past" (Norcross, 2005). The disadvantage associated with this approach, and one the NCLT addresses, is that there may not be a clear conceptual framework describing how techniques drawn from divergent theories go together.

The Problems with Eclecticism

The most persistent criticism level against the practice of eclecticism is that it completely ignores theory. In addition to ignoring theory, there is a de-emphasis on any research basis for the various combined approaches.

Another of the major issues taken with eclecticism is that the combination of therapeutic approaches selected by the therapist is often without conventions or rules dictating how or which theories were combined. As a result, eclectic practice is often idiosyncratic with various practitioners picking therapeutic approaches based on preference or past training as opposed to any scientific model as to what might work best in a particular situation. Selections are often made on the basis of what the therapist might feel comfortable in performing.

Integrative Approaches

Integrative approaches blend elements from different models of psychotherapy to form a new whole. There is a clear distinction between integrative and eclectic approaches in that integration suggests that the elements are part of one combined approach to theory and practice, as opposed to eclecticism which draws idiosyncratically from several approaches in the approach to a particular case (Woolfe & Palmer, 2000).

In fact, in practice most therapists practice what has become known as assimilative integration. Therapists are trained in, and often select a primary theoretical orientation as a foundation, but then incorporate ideas and strategies from other sources into their practice (Messer, Norcross, Goldfried, & Messer, 1992).

Integrating Psychotherapy Techniques

Some attempts to create a unifying model for eclectic approaches have centered on the elements that constitute the therapy relationship, particularly the methods and techniques common to all forms of psychotherapy including catharsis, conditioning, confrontation, desensitization, empathy, extinction, genuineness, immediacy, insight, interpretation, listening, placebos, probing, reinforcement, reflection, resistance, respect, shaping, silence, and transference (Patterson, 1985). Eclectic models such as integrative therapy (Norcross, 2005) systematically matches evidence-based treatment methods and healing relationships to the client on the basis of multiple diagnostic features, including stage of change, reactance level, culture, and preferences. These approaches have been labeled common factors approaches.

In 1991, Lazarus argued that not only has theoretical integration failed to provide greater consensus or any data-based treatment combinations, but that a state of even greater chaos now prevailed, and argued for a technical eclecticism grounded in observation rather than theory. Messer argued that all observation is informed by theory, and that techniques selectively imported from other therapies must be assimilated to the new contexts and be validated through clinical use and experimentation (Lazarus & Messer, 1991).

Elements of Another Way: Memory Reconsolidation at the Level of the Synapse

The above state of affairs changed dramatically when three independent groups of researchers converged on the conclusion that a wide variety of different psychotherapies can be integrated via their common ability to trigger the neurobiological mechanism of memory reconsolidation in such a way as to lead to deconsolidation of a previously learned emotional response (Ecker, Ticic, & Hulley, 2013). To be clear, it is not the memory per se that is affected. Rather, it is the emotional memory that is under discussion. The episodic memory for the event will not be erased. It is the pairing between the memory and the emotional response that will be altered.

Prior to this research the prevailing wisdom was that learning that occurs in the presence of strong emotion becomes locked permanently into subcortical implicit

Table 3.1 Disorders whose symptomology are alleviated by memory reconsolidation

Attention deficit/hyperactivity disorder	Anxiety	Anger
Attachment disorder	Compulsive behavior	Depression
Guilt	Low arousal	Low motivation
Low self worth	Poor motivation	Post-traumatic stress disorder
Perfectionism	Panic attacks	Phobic responses

memory circuits by special synapses, never to be unlocked. Researchers, for the first time, had been able to activate a learned emotional (targeted emotional learning) response and under certain conditions found that its previously locked neural circuit had temporarily shifted back into an unlocked, de-consolidated, labile, destabilized, or plastic state, which allowed the emotional learning to be completely nullified, along with behavioral responses it had been driving. The temporarily labile circuit soon consolidates once again, returning it to a locked condition, which is why researchers named this newly discovered type of neuroplasticity memory reconsolidation. Based on this research, it is clear that the consolidation of emotional learning or emotional memory is not a one-time, finite process resulting in indelible emotional learning. Clinically speaking, counteracting and regulating unwanted acquired responses, through, for example, relaxation is not necessarily the way to address these emotional issues. Relearning the response, or emotional pairing, is.

NCLT is designed to reteach emotional responses using well-established principles of learning working in conjunction with empirically valid therapeutic techniques. As such, it represents a truly integrated approach that is based not on features of the therapeutic endeavor, but on the known science as regard neuropsychology, neuroplasticity, neurophysiology, and learning.

Research has identified a number of clinical conditions whose symptomology is alleviated by memory reconsolidation that occurs as part of NCLT Table 3.1.

Requirements for De-consolidation: Reactivation Plus Mismatch

In order for the memories associated with emotional respondency to be de-consolidated, a critical experience must take place when the emotional memory and related behavioral response are reactivated (Pedreira, Perez-Cuesta, & Maldonado, 2004). This second experience consists of perceptions that sharply mismatch, or deviate substantially from what the reactivated target memory expects and predicts about how the world functions. Clinically, the mismatch can be either a full contradiction or disconfirmation of the target memory, or a novel, salient variation relative to the target memory. On the other hand, if the target memory is reactivated by familiar cues but not concurrently mismatched, synapses do not unlock and reconsolidation is not induced (Hernandez & Kelley, 2004).

Therapeutically, a three step process is initially required in order to carry out the transformation sequence identified in reconsolidation research:

1. Symptom identification. Actively clarify with the client what to regard as the presenting symptom(s). These include the specific behaviors, somatics, emotions, and/or thoughts that the client wants to eliminate and when they happen. This includes the percepts and contexts that evoke or intensify them.
2. Retrieval of target learning into explicit awareness, as a visceral emotional experience, the details of the emotional learning or schema underlying and driving the presenting symptom.
3. Identification of disconfirming knowledge. Identify a vivid experience (past or present) that can serve as living knowledge that is fundamentally incompatible with the model of reality in the target emotional learning in step A, such that both cannot possibly be true. The disconfirming material may or may not be appealing to the client as being more "positive" or preferred; what matters is that it be mutually exclusive with the target learning. It may be already part of the client's personal knowledge or may be created by a new experience.

There is a fourth step wherein the client verifies the new emotional response by generalizing it into new situations and contexts (Ecker et al., 2013).

NCLT and Memory Reconciliation

The above sequence of steps is entirely consistent with NCLT practice as described in our book on the research justification for NCLT (Wasserman & Wasserman, 2016). As does NCLT, memory reconciliation models have a learning-based model for the therapeutic enterprise. "New learning always creates new neural circuits, but transformational change occurs only when new learning radically unlearns, unwires and replaces an existing learning, rather than merely forming alongside existing learning and competitively regulating it. The use of new learning to erase an existing, unwanted learning is precisely what the therapeutic reconsolidation process achieves. It consists of steps that guide therapy yet allow an extremely broad range of techniques to be used for guiding the key experiences, so a therapist's individual style of working continues to have great scope of expression" (Ecker et al., 2013, p. 95).

NCLT Is an Integrative Therapeutic Model

The NCLT model easily fits within the group of models described as compliant with the memory reconciliation framework. This group includes accelerated experiential dynamic psychotherapy, coherence therapy (formerly depth oriented brief therapy), eye movement desensitization and reprocessing (EMDR), emotion-focused therapy (EFT), focusing-oriented psychotherapy, interpersonal neurobiology (IPNB), neuro-linguistic programming (NLP), and traumatic incident reduction (TIR) to name a few (Ecker et al., 2013). NCLT practice permits the inclusion of many techniques as long as those techniques utilize the laws of learning to effect predictable changes to the client's connectome as regards neural learning.

NCLT Integrates All Other Models

While it might be tempting to think of NCLT as just another integrative model, there is a striking and profound difference between NCLT and these other models. NCLT posits exactly how and why changes occur and connects those changes to the individual's neurobiology. This is different from other models. For example consider this statement from the EMDR International Association: "No one knows how any form of psychotherapy works neurobiologically or in the brain." However, we do know that when a person is very upset, their brain cannot process information as it does ordinarily. One moment becomes "frozen in time," and remembering a trauma may feel as bad as going through it the first time because the images, sounds, smells, and feelings haven't changed. Such memories have a lasting negative effect that interferes with the way a person sees the world and the way they relate to other people. EMDR seems to have a direct effect on the way that the brain processes information. Normal information processing is resumed, so following a successful EMDR session, a person no longer relives the images, sounds, and feelings when the event is brought to mind. You still remember what happened, but it is less upsetting (EMDR International Association, 2014). This position is not sufficient for the development of a science of psychotherapy. The objective of any integrative system of psychotherapy must include the philosophical and theoretical foundations, the derivative principles guiding practice and methods to implement the practice (Patterson, 2000).

NCLT knows exactly why and how the desired changes are occurring and what is more describes the steps necessary to make these changes in a manner that is consistent with how the brain processes information. It incorporates the memory reconciliation research with known models of learning to produce a comprehensive framework that may logically include any empirically valid technique designed to produce a specific learning/behavioral sequence. The core constructs of NCLT are empirically verifiable and although as yet there is no research on the NCLT model per se, there is a long history of research, amply documented in *Depathologizing Psychopathology* (2016), that thoroughly documents the validity of its component parts. NCLT is a model that articulates how change occurs in therapy and as a result can be the basis of a scientifically responsible integration of psychotherapy practice. It is therefore more than a new type of therapy. It is an organizational structure for all therapy, organized around solid science relating evidence-based practice based upon how the brain processes information.

References

Ecker, B., Ticic, R., & Hulley, L. (2013). A primer on memory reconsolidation and its psychotherapeutic use as a core process of profound change. *Neuropsychotherapist, 1*, 82–88. doi:10.12744/tnpt(1)082-099.

EMDR International Association. (2014). *How does EMDR work.* Retrieved from EMDRIA: https://emdria.site-ym.com/?119

Grohol, J. (2015, April). *Types of therapies: Theoretical orientations and practices of therapists.* Retrieved from *PsychCentral*: http://psychcentral.com/therapy.htm

Hernandez, P., & Kelley, A. (2004). Long-term memory for instrumental responses does not undergo protein synthesis-dependent reconsolidation upon retrieval. *Learning & Memory, 11*, 748–754. doi:10.1101/lm.84904.

Lazarus, A., & Messer, S. (1991). Does chaos prevail? An exchange on technical eclecticism and assimilative integration. *Journal of Psychotherapy Integration, 1*(2), 143–158. doi:10.1037/h0101225.

Messer, S. (1992). A critical examination of belief structures in integrative and eclectic psychotherapy. In J. Norcross, & M. Goldfried, Messer, S. B.. Handbook of psychotherapy integration. (pp. 130-165). New York: Basic Books.

Norcross, J. (2005). A primer on psychotherapy integration. In J. Norcross & M. Goldfried (Eds.), *Handbook of psychotherapy integration* (2nd ed., pp. 3–23). New York: Oxford University Press.

Patterson, C. (1985). *The therapeutic relationship: Foundations for an eclectic psychotherapy.* Belmont, CA: Thomson Brooks/Cole Publishing.

Patterson, C. (2000). Eclecticism in psychotherapy: Is integration possible. In C. Patterson (Ed.), *Understanding psychotherapy: 50 years of client centered theory and practice* (pp. 157–161). Ross-on-Wye, UK: PCCS Books.

Pedreira, M., Perez-Cuesta, L., & Maldonado, H. (2004). Mismatch between what is expected and what actually occurs triggers memory reconsolidation or extinction. *Learning & Memory, 11*, 579–585. doi:10.1101/lm.76904.

Wasserman, T., & Wasserman, L. (2016). *Depathologizing psychopathology.* New York: Springer.

Woolfe, R., & Palmer, S. (2000). *Integrative and eclectic counselling and psychotherapy.* London/Thousand Oaks, CA: Sage Publications.

Chapter 4
NCLT and Life Course Theory

A careful reading of what we have written about the nature of mental illness here and in the past (Wasserman & Wasserman, 2016) would suggest that NCLT would support a model that would propose that mental illness was as much acquired as it was caused. The model we would support would have a number of properties, but chief among them would be the idea that multiple variables and life experiences interacted with a constitutionally provided core to produce an outcome that is sometimes healthy and adaptive, such as resilience and, as in the case of mental illness, sometimes not adaptive. There is broadening support for this model. For example, The World Health Organization, in its summary report entitled *Promoting Mental Health* (World Health Organization, 2004), noted that "mental health and mental illness are determined by multiple and interacting social, psychological, and biological factors, just as health and illness in general" (p. 12). In other words, the same variables promote either mental health or illness depending upon how they impact the individual's developing system. In fact, there is just such a model available that recognizes and embraces these concepts, and that as applied to issues of mental health by extension, is consistent with, and applicable to NCLT theory because it looks at the totality of a person in the complexity of their environment and experiences. It is called Life course theory.

Life Course Theory

Life course theory (LCT) is a conceptual model that attempts to explain health and disease development and disparity across populations and over time. It is intended as an epidemiological model as opposed to a medical model of disease causation, and focuses on groups as opposed to individuals (Fine & Kotelchuck, 2010). LCT focuses on differences in health patterns as a result of broad social, economic, and environmental factors as underlying causes of persistent inequalities in health for a wide range of diseases and conditions across population groups. LCT is also

© Springer International Publishing AG 2017
T. Wasserman, L.D. Wasserman, *Neurocognitive Learning Therapy: Theory and Practice*, DOI 10.1007/978-3-319-60849-5_4

community (or "place") focused, since social, economic, and environmental patterns are closely linked to community and neighborhood settings.

LCT is also applied more widely in a positive, or health oriented manner by attempting to understand factors that can help all people achieve optimal health and developmental trajectories over a lifetime, and even inter-generationally. Specific to the issue of health, LCT seeks to identify the factors that influence the capacity of individuals or populations to reach their full potential for health and well-being.

LCT is based upon several key concepts:

Pathways or Trajectories

Health pathways or trajectories are developed and constructed, or deconstructed, over the course of a lifetime. Patterns can be amalgamated and predicted for populations and communities based on social, economic, and environmental exposures and experiences. Individual trajectories within those community patterns may vary. An individual's life course does not reflect a series of discrete steps, but rather an ongoing and ever reintegrating continuum of exposures, experiences, and interactions.

Early Programming

Early experiences, as much as and perhaps to a greater extent than later experiences, can facilitate the development of specific pathways and trajectories, and significantly influence an individual's future health and development. NCLT posits that this is because these early experiences form the basis of early automated routines upon which the more complex adult routines are based. The early experiences include everything from prenatal programming (i.e., exposure in utero) to intergenerational programming (i.e., the health of the mother prior to conception) that impact the health of the baby and developing child. LCT modeling suggests that these early experiences and related automated response routines can result in adverse programming, resulting directly in a disease or condition, or making an individual more vulnerable or susceptible to developing a disease or condition in the future.

Critical or Sensitive Periods

In line with developmental theory (Piaget & Inhelder, 1972) this concept posits that while adverse events and exposures can have an impact at any point in a person's life course, their impact is greatest at specific critical or sensitive periods of development (e.g., during fetal development, in early childhood, and during adolescence).

Cumulative Impact

Cumulative experiences ("learning" in NCLT terminology) programs ("automates" in NCLT terminology) an individual's future health and development. As a mental health example, LCT would conjecture that while individual episodes of stress may have minimal impact on an individual's otherwise positive mental health trajectory, the cumulative impact of multiple stresses over time may have a profound, negative and direct impact on health and development, as well as an indirect impact via associated behavioral or health service seeking changes.

Risk and Protective Factors

Over the course of a lifetime certain protective factors improve health and contribute to healthy development, while certain risk factors diminish health and make it more difficult to reach full developmental potential. Thus, pathways are multi-determined, and the results idiosyncratic to the development of the individual. There is a wide range of both risk and protective factors that are not limited to individual behavioral patterns or receipt (or lack) of things like nutrition, medical care, and social services, but also include factors related to family, neighborhood, community, and social policy. Examples of protective factors include, among others, a nurturing family, a safe neighborhood, strong and positive relationships, economic security, access to quality primary care and other health services, and access to high quality schools and early care and education. Examples of risk factors include, among others, food insecurity, homelessness, living in poverty, unsafe neighborhoods, domestic violence, environmental pollution, inadequate education opportunities, racial discrimination, being born low birth weight, and lack of access to quality health services.

Fine and Kotelchuck (2010) summarized and simplified the four key life course concepts as the following:

Timeline: Today's experiences and exposures influence tomorrow's health.

Timing: Health trajectories are particularly affected during critical or sensitive periods.

Environment: The broader community environment—biologic, physical, and social—strongly affects the capacity to be healthy.

Equity: While genetic make-up offers both protective and risk factors for disease conditions, inequality in health reflects more than genetics and personal choice.

Life Course Theory and Mental Health

A life course model for the development of disorders of mental health is concerned with the interaction of social and biological factors in the production of mental illness over the life span from the postnatal period to old age, as noted by Koenen, Rudenstine, Susser, and Galea (2013). They note increasing evidence that mental disorders, previously perceived to emerge in adulthood, may have their origins early in life. A central premise of the life course model, as it pertains to mental health, might be paraphrased as follows; changing behaviors alters trajectory (Elder, 1998).

Elder's (1998) work gives a clearer picture of the complex interactions that might be considered within an LCT-based model. For example, he reported on work that viewed the family, and how it adapted to the circumstances that impinged upon it, "as a central link between a generalized economic decline and the well-being of children. Poverty indebtedness, income loss, and unstable work increased the felt economic pressure of families. The stronger this reported pressure, the greater the risk of depressed feelings and marital negativity among parents. These processes tended to undermine nurturant parenting, and increased the likelihood of emotional distress, academic trouble, and problem behavior among boys and girls" (p. 2).

NCLT and Life Course Theory

The epidemiology of mental illness according to the life course model considers the interaction of a multiplicity of factors within a population-based context, with specific focus on its relevance to public health. NCLT takes this population focus and extends the model down to the individual client. For example, each of the family- or community-based factors that Elder (1998) identifies as affecting the family, affects each and every member of the family idiosyncratically. After all, some family members may adapt, while others fail to adapt. As Elder puts it, the life course "principle of human agency states that individuals construct their own life course through the choices and actions they take within the opportunities and constraints of history and social circumstances" (p. 4).

NCLT extends this model to the treatment of mental illness, conceptualized as emerging as a result of life course processes. Its focus is on the individual, and how that individual adapts to the life course events with which they interact. Each of the factors impinging on an individual represents an opportunity for that individual to derive some knowledge from that experience. That knowledge is based on what has come before and is filtered by an established lens. The knowledge, lens and response that is established for that experience, develops into automatic patterns of response and related emotions. Some of these patterns of response are maladaptive. It is those automated maladaptive and individualized responses that are the targets of therapeutic intervention.

Therapy as a Turning Point

Life course modeling hypothesizes that there are points in time when an event or circumstance alters the trajectory of a pathway. These points in time are called turning points (Teruya & Hser, 2010). "A turning point often involves a particular event, experience, or awareness that results in changes in the direction of a pathway, or persistent trajectory over the long-term" (p. 89). The term, turning point, has typically been used in conjunction with certain life events. Not all events or experiences lead to changes in life trajectories. Only those events that redirect paths are considered turning points in life. Turning points are determined in hind sight, as it is only with the passing of a period of time that the stability of the redirected pathway can be confirmed.

For some people, turning points may be the result of single dramatic events that bring about abrupt changes (Elder, Gimbel, & Ivie, 1991). For others, changes are more incremental, occurring gradually over time (Pickles & Rutter, 1991) and accumulate whereby at some point, an "epiphany" triggers a decision to radically change one's life. For us, this is a description of the NCLT process. It is a series of planned events that evoke emotionally based patterns of responses and their associated behaviors that cause a change in the client's life course towards a more adaptive lifestyle.

Examples of the Interplay Between Life Course Theory and NCLT Treatment

Depression

The life course model and treatment approaches derived from it are well suited for understanding depression. This is because causation in depression clearly appears to be multifactorial. These factors include interactions between genes and stressful events, the development of the connectome, the presence or absence of early life trauma, and the interaction of early life trauma with later stress in life. In addition to causation, the timing of onset and remission of depression varies widely, suggesting differing trajectories of symptoms over long periods of time. All of this strongly indicates that there are likely differing causes and differing outcomes, with early life events and development appearing to be important risk factors for depression. These early life events include exposure to acute and chronic stress in the first years of life (Colman & Ataullahjan, 2010). In a similar vein, Beck and others have proposed a comparable multifaceted model of the genesis of depression, stating that their newly developed unified model is based on the premise that depression represents "an adaptation to the perceived loss of essential human resources that provides access to the necessities of life including the loss of a family member, a romantic partner, or a peer group. To individuals who are at greater risk for severe depression because of specific genetic or environmental factors, this loss is more likely to be viewed as devastating and insurmountable" (Beck & Bredemeier, 2016, p. 1).

NCLT treatment is based on a similar understanding of the multifactorial nature of the etiology of depression; one that includes genetic, connectomic, and environmental factors. NCLT would look at the responses to many of those factors as learned combinations of emotional, physiological, and behavioral responses that represent the targets for treatment. While the model would understand the trajectory that led the individual to respond in a manner that generated behaviors consistent with a diagnosis of depression, it would not consider those responses predetermined, totally predictable, or immutable to change. On the contrary, it would consider the amalgam of responses that constituted the outcome as one possible, and indeed idiosyncratic, adaptive outcome. It would understand that other outcomes were just as likely and possible. The model would also understand that the preferred and automated outcome was not immutable, because altering the response set is also possible. Depression in this view, for many people, becomes a state not a trait. It can be altered by changing the characteristics of response sets utilizing the techniques described elsewhere in this volume.

Attention Deficit Hyperactivity Disorder

There are also life course model considerations for disorders of emotional regulation such as in ADHD. Wilens and Spenser (2010) note that treatment requires consideration of all aspects of an individual's life, and should be multimodal treatment including educational, family, and individual support. Thus, while a disorder such as ADHD has a presumably strong neurobiological core, the patterns of disruptive learned behavior and emotional response extend into every area of an individual's life (Bernfort, Nordfelt, & Perrsson, 2008) and need to be addressed in successful treatment. Perhaps to belabor, but surely emphasize the point NCLT and life course models stress, that individuals build their response patterns upon their constitutionally derived connectomics, and it is these response patterns that are the target for treatment.

Anxiety-Based Disorders

Similarly, there are significant Life Course Framework implications in the epidemiology of anxiety disorders. For example, in a meta-analysis of studies examining the heterogeneity or homogeneity of anxiety in either the nature of symptoms experienced, or in patterns of symptoms over time (labeled symptom trajectories), Nandi, Beard, and Galea (2009) found growing evidence for mood and anxiety disorders being differentiable by both symptom syndromes and trajectories. Factors associated with these disorders varied between these subtypes. It was not clear whether this finding of symptom subtypes (trajectory subtypes) represented a causal pathway influenced by either genetic or environmental factors. NCLT postulates that these trajectories represent the accumulated learning experience of the individual in reaction to the environmental exigencies that the individual has experienced.

In summary, there is a good deal of overlap between the life course framework and NCLT models in terms of the etiology and epidemiology of disorders of mental health. While the life course framework largely concerns itself with the predictive epidemiological factors, the NCLT model emphasizes the treatment aspects of what is a multifactorial model of the development and manifestation of disorders of mental health.

References

Beck, A., & Bredemeier, K. (2016). A unified model of depression: Integrating clinical, cognitive, biological, and evolutionary perspectives. *Clinical Psychological Science*. Advance online publication. doi:10.1177/2167702616628523.

Bernfort, L., Nordfelt, S., & Perrsson, J. (2008). ADHD from a socio-economic perspective. *Acta Paediatrica, 97*(2), 239–245. doi:10.1111/j.1651-2227.2007.00611.x.

Colman, J., & Ataullahjan, A. (2010). Life course perspectives on the epidemiology of depression. *Canadian Journal of Psychiatry, 55*(10), 622–632.

Elder, G. (1998). The life course as developmental theory. *Child Development, 69*(1), 1–12.

Elder, G., Gimbel, C., & Ivie, R. (1991). Turning points in life: The case of military service and war. *Military Psychology, 3*, 215–231.

Fine, A., & Kotelchuck, M. (2010, November). *Rethinking MCH: The life course model as an organizing framework*. Retrieved from mchb.hrsa.gov: http://mchb.hrsa.gov/lifecourse/rethinkingmchlifecourse.pdf

Koenen, K., Rudenstine, D., Susser, E., & Galea, S. (2013). *A life course approach to mental disorders*. Oxford: Oxford University Press.

Nandi, A., Beard, J., & Galea, S. (2009). Epidemiologic heterogeneity of common mood and anxiety disorders over the lifecourse in the general population: A systematic review. *BMC Psychiatry, 9*, 31. doi:10.1186/1471-244X-9-31.

Piaget, J., & Inhelder, B. (1972). *The psychology of the child*. London: Routledge.

Pickles, A., & Rutter, M. (1991). Statistical and conceptual models of 'turning points' in developmental processes. In D. Magnusson, L. Bergman, G. Rudinger, & B. Torestad (Eds.), *Problems and methods in longitudinal research: Stability and change* (pp. 133–165). Cambridge, UK: Cambridge University Press.

Teruya, C., & Hser, Y. (2010). Turning points in the life course: Current findings and future directions in drug use research. *Current Drug Abuse Review, 3*(3), 189–195.

Wasserman, T., & Wasserman, L. (2016). *Depathologizing psychopathology*. New York: Springer.

Wilens, T., & Spenser, T. (2010). Understanding attention-deficit/hyperactivity disorder from childhood to adulthood. *Postgraduate Medicine, 122*(5), 97–109. doi:10.3810/pgm.2010.09.2206.

World Health Organization. (2004). *Promoting mental health*. Geneva, Switzerland: World Health Organization.

Chapter 5
Reward Recognition in NCLT Practice

People make decisions all the time. By decisions we do not only mean complex decisions such as for whom one should vote, or whether man is inherently good. There are more mundane decisions about what to have for dinner, or whether or not to see a particular movie. We make decisions about whether or not to cross a particular street to get to a destination, whether to pick up a blue pen or a red pen, and which canape to select from a tray of identical canapes. In fact, we make decisions every waking minute.

Estimates vary, but it has been suggested that human adults make 35,000 remotely conscious decisions each day. Assuming 16 waking hours each day, that's almost 2200 decisions every hour, 36 decisions every minute and 1 decision about every one and a half seconds. Research has suggested that we make more than 220 decisions each day on just food alone (Wansink & Sobol, 2007). Young children make as few as 3000 decisions in a day. The more than tenfold increase in decision load on the human system as we reach adulthood reflects the increasingly complex, choice rich, environment most adults find themselves in as a part of everyday living.

Decisions simply represent choices between two or more options. Each decision is not an isolated instance. The effect of decisions compound one upon the other. These compounded decisions not only build upon each other, they act interdependently with other contextually relevant decisions, resulting in a complex web of interconnected patterns of actions and emotional responses. Some decisions are practiced so much that they become automatic; we do them without having to think about them. This is a critical point. Decisions require cognitive effort. The goal of most human thinking, however, is to preserve limited cognitive effort capacity for critical and novel situations (Bettman, Johnson, & Payne, 1990). For example, think about your weekly trip to the grocery store. If you have lived in a particular location for a while, the decisions made as part of that trip have been organized into a sequence, and have been practiced many times. These decisions include the best

© Springer International Publishing AG 2017
T. Wasserman, L.D. Wasserman, *Neurocognitive Learning Therapy: Theory and Practice*, DOI 10.1007/978-3-319-60849-5_5

route to travel, the lane to be in, and whether to turn left, right, or go straight at certain intersections. After some practice, we no longer think about them individually, they automatically occur in a sequence. Those of us who drive have each had the experience wherein we are driving a well-rehearsed route and suddenly become alert: Perhaps a new building has been erected, or a tree removed giving us an unfamiliar view. We all say rhetorically that "we have been driving on automatic." In fact, we have. We have all been "saving" our cognitive resources to apply to a more critical or novel situation, perhaps what we anticipate once we reach our destination, or perhaps a professional or domestic issue.

Canon-Bard Theory of Emotion and NCLT

Building networks of decisions that work together, mostly in an automatic manner, is the continuing work of a lifetime. These networks of decisions are developed to take us to various outcomes. These outcomes can include patterns of behavior and patterns of emotional responses. These decision-making processes may reflect choices made between two solely independent neutral stimuli, or reflect choices made between stimuli that have previously produced visceral responses to their appearance. In the latter case, follow-up choices may reflect established conditioned responses. To this extent the NCLT model of emotional response is related to the Canon-Bard model (and its progeny) (Papez, 1937). This theory posits that people simultaneously experience emotions and physiological reactions. Essentially, their hypothesis is that emotions result when brain systems, such as the thalamus, signals a response to a stimulus. Among other things, the thalamus influences motor control, auditory or visual signals, and the sending of sensory signals. The end result is the physiological reaction. For example, if you see a spider, you may become afraid, and at the same time, you may scream or tremble. Essentially, these models posit that an external stimulus activates receptors, and this excitation starts impulses toward the cortex. Upon arriving in the cortex, the impulses are associated with learned processes that determine the direction of the subsequent response.

These patterns of end stage behaviors and emotions are idiosyncratic. Each individual, by dint of their environmental interactions with their connectome, are unique in the behavioral and emotional patterns they develop. There is recent research that clearly demonstrates that there are powerful learned influences of culture on the core expressions of emotion that were once, incorrectly, considered biologically hardwired (Jack, Garrod, Yu, Caldara, & Schyns, 2012). This, then again, suggests the effects of learning on the connectome.

Decision-Making Models, the Importance of Reward, and NCLT

As might be expected, there are several theoretical models that have been used to represent the human decision-making process. While a discussion of these models is beyond the scope of this book, a brief review of the model used in formulating NCLT principles will provide a useful backdrop to the discussion as to the utility of understanding the importance of reward valuation in NCLT clinical practice.

Reward valuation is the process by which we calculate the probability and benefits of a prospective outcome. We engage in this process all of the time. We calculate and decide just how desirable something is. We assess how likely it is that we will be able to get what we want. These processes may include references to accumulated or to new information, to social context, and/or to prior experience. This valuation is influenced by prior learning, memory, current physical states, etc. As an example, we might be determining the reward value of a master degree or Ph.D. We would consider the prestige and utility of each degree. We might call upon what we previously believed about each degree. We might consider the cost of each degree. We might take into account just how fatigued we are after a shift at our current job and the likelihood of being able to apply ourselves to studying for a degree.

NCLT describes the choice making process using a sequential sampling model for multi-attribute binary choice options, called multiattribute attention switching (MAAS) model as the basis of its understanding of reward valuation (Diederich & Oswald, 2014). When a person is confronted by making a choice between two or more stimuli, this model assumes a separate sampling process for each attribute of each of the available choices. That is, when we are thinking about deciding between choices, our attention switches from one attribute consideration to the next. The order in which attributes are considered, as well as for how long each attribute is considered (attention time), influences the predicted choice probabilities and choice response times. Both order of attribute consideration and attention time given to each attribute are important targets for discussion within an NCLT session. As a point of reference, think about your teenaged client deciding between tackling his history essay or playing the latest video game.

It is often the case that individuals emphasize differing aspects of their desired choice. It is also true that oft times some people prefer attributes that other people would de-emphasize. In this way depressed individuals might value the amount of energy not expended to complete a task as the most important attribute to consider. Although that sounds awkward, how many times have you had a client express "I can't. I just don't have the energy." Other times patients tend to give very short consideration to attributes that most people would think more carefully about. In this way, impulsive individuals can be noted to select and begin tasks without proper planning or consideration of the consequences. Offering examples of teenagers making impulsive decisions based upon only one aspect of reward valuation would require its own book.

Sequential sampling models assume several things that are necessary for their operation. Given that MAAS is a mathematical model, the first assumption is that stimulus and choice alternative characteristics can be mapped onto a hypothetical numerical value representing the instantaneous level of evidence or preference. The second is that some random fluctuation of this value over time occurs. Finally, these models assume that evidence is accumulated over time, and that a final choice is made as soon as the evidence reaches a critical threshold. Given that humans are not computers, the factors within each of these assumptions will vary by individual.

While not a part of MAAS modeling, NCLT further assumes that these choice decisions, if confronted frequently enough, can become automated.

Cue Competition, Blocking, and NCLT

The effect of automaticity and the pre-learned often maladaptive responses seen in treatment can best be understood when you understand the concepts of cue competition and blocking. In the cognitive psychology literature on decision making, cue competition occurs when alternative cues compete to gain associative predictiveness of the outcome. Associative predictiveness means which cues are associated, through learning, with which outcomes. There are two elements to consider. One is the degree to which an individual's attention is determined by exploiting what is known about the most valid predictors of outcomes. The second element consists of those stimuli that are associated with the greatest degree of uncertainty about subsequent events (Beesley, Nguyen, Pearson, & Le Pelley, 2015). This ongoing cue competition is fundamental in associative learning (Kruschke, 2001).

Blocking is part of a group of effects that are associated with the concept of cue competition. These effects, typically termed "cue competition" effects, define how cue competition operates in human learning situations. Common amongst all cue competition effects is that a cue-outcome relation is poorly learned, or poorly expressed, because the cue is trained in the presence of an alternative predictor or cause of the outcome. In blocking, the cue of interest is trained in compound with a competing cue that was previously paired with the outcome. The effect of the competing previously trained cue is to block the new cue from stimulating the outcome (Boddez, Haesen, Baeyens, & Beckers, 2014). Simply stated, old responses block the learning and application of new responses. In treatment, this implies that old, automated, maladaptive behavioral responses will effectively block the learning and acquisition of new more adaptive responses. These blocks are also targets of intervention in NCLT-based treatment. The blocks must be identified as such, and systematically removed, utilizing the learning processes outlined elsewhere in this volume.

The Relationship of Rewards and Decision Making

As we have pointed out, perceived rewards are critical and involved in all learning, approach behavior, choices, and emotions. Central to the utility of such learning in a therapeutic context is our ability to first neurophysiologically represent, and then clinically understand the value of rewarding and punishing stimuli, establish predictions of when and where such rewards and punishments will occur, and use those predictions to form the basis of decisions that guide behavior. There are structures, including the ventromedial prefrontal cortex (encompassing orbital and medial prefrontal regions), amygdala, striatum, and dopaminergic midbrain that are highly interconnected, and together, can be considered as an integrated reward recognition network (O'Doherty, 2004).

A Brief Detour to the Neuroanatomy of Reward Representation

One component of the reward network, in particular for coding for stimulus reward value, is the orbitofrontal cortex (OFC). Human neuroimaging studies have confirmed a role for human OFC in coding stimulus value from a variety of sensory modalities, including such primary ones as taste, olfaction, somatosensory, auditory, and vision as well as for more complex rewards such as money (O'Doherty, 2004).

It is quite obvious that it is advantageous to be able to predict in advance when and where rewards or punishments will occur so that behavior can be planned appropriately. Neuroimaging studies have implicated amygdala, OFC, and ventral striatum in reward prediction (O'Doherty, 2004).

The ability to form predictions of reward is only part of the process of deciding. It is also required that the person be able to act on those predictions. In a given situation, specific intermediate actions might need to be performed to obtain reward. This requires the learning of stimulus–response, or response–reward associations. The dorsal striatum has been implicated as involved in creation of such a contingency that is established between responses and reward (O'Doherty, 2004).

Decision Making

"To choose between different actions it is necessary to maintain a representation of the predicted future reward associated with each action. Such predictions then need to be compared and evaluated to select the action with the highest overall predicted reward value. This process is more complicated than at first sight, because estimations of predicted reward vary in their quality and depend on the number of samples of that action in the past as well as the variance of the reward distribution" (O'Doherty, 2004, p. 773). Research has identified a role of the OFC in these processes.

Reward and Decision-Making Network

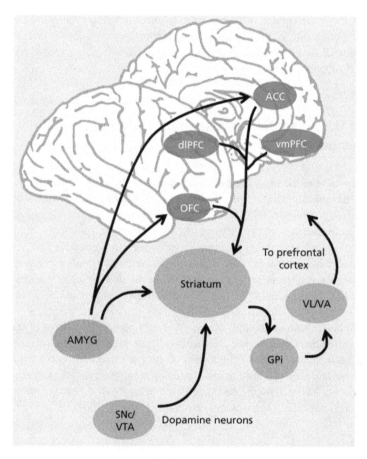

This reward-related learning function is mediated by neuronal reward prediction error signals which implement basic constructs of reinforcement learning theory (Schultz, 2015). Neurophysiologically, reward signals are found in dopamine neurons, which emit a global reward signal to striatum and frontal cortex, and in specific neurons in striatum, amygdala, and frontal cortex projecting to select neuronal populations. The approach and choice decision functions involve a subjective determination of value, which are objectively assessed by behavioral choices, eliciting internal, subjective reward preferences.

Deciding About Reward in the Future

When humans are offered the choice between rewards available at different points in time, the relative values of the options are discounted according to their expected delays until delivery. Actually, two separate systems are recruited depending on the immediacy of each choice. For rewards that are immediately available, parts of the limbic system associated with the midbrain dopamine system, including paralimbic cortex, are preferentially activated. When delay of reward is involved, regions of the lateral prefrontal cortex and posterior parietal cortex are recruited. Interestingly, the amount of relative engagement of the two systems is directly related to subject choice, with greater relative fronto-parietal activity occurring when subjects choose longer term options (McClure, Laibson, Lowenstein, & Cohen, 2004).

It was initially assumed that the delay in reward valence that occurred over time was both uniform and time dependent. More recent research indicates that this is not the case. Three different, sometimes competing, mechanisms that are implemented in the brain, representation, anticipation, and self-control are all factors in determining reward strength of future reward strength (Berns, Lainson, & Lowenstein, 2007). There are other factors as well, that are based at least in part, on these core three. For example, a major factor influencing utility is uncertainty. In individuals termed "risk averse," uncertainty reduces the utility of a reward (a reward has less value if I am afraid that I won't get it), whereas individuals termed "risk seekers" find higher reward possibilities in an uncertain reward.

These findings have important consideration for clinical practice in that they indicate that those with either poor self-control or high expectation will value the future reward differently than an individual for whom these circumstances did not exist. For example, there is research that suggests that impulsive individuals weight time differently, thereby imposing a higher cost of waiting. As a result, impulsive individuals overestimate the duration of time intervals and, as a consequence, discount the value of delayed rewards more strongly than do self-controlled individuals (Wittman & Paulus, 2008). In addition, dysfunctional reward processing, accompanied by a limited ability to tolerate reward delays, has been proposed as an important feature in attention-deficit/hyperactivity disorder (ADHD) (Pichta et al., 2009).

Individuals are often required to make choices between an alternative with higher overall value and a more initially tempting, but ultimately lesser option. These issues are often the ones that confront us in therapy. There are multiple examples. Should I flirt with the attractive person or remain faithful to my spouse? Should I gamble the rent money? Should I do my homework or play my video game? Should I take the adjustable rate mortgage even though I may not be able to afford the payment that will be required 2 years from now? In these situations, and many more, the individuals we see often make the impulsive, immediate choice. They do not delay gratification, or in NCLT terms, they do not correctly value the distant rewards. We have written extensively on the role of reward valuation in individuals with attention deficit disorder (Wasserman & Wasserman, 2015). Therapy is always about decision making, and optimal decision making requires self-control.

There is a neurobiology of self-control. Goal-directed decisions have their basis in a common value signal encoded in ventromedial prefrontal cortex (vmPFC), and exercising self-control involves the modulation of this value signal by dorsolateral prefrontal cortex (DLPFC) (Hare, Camerer, & Rangel, 2009).

The Relationship of Reward Decision Making and Emotion

The somatic marker hypothesis (Bechara, Damasio, & Demasio, 2000) provides a systems-level neuroanatomical and cognitive model for decision making, and the influence on it by emotion. This model posits that decision making is a process that is influenced by marker signals that arise in bio-regulatory processes, including those that express themselves in emotions and feelings. The influence of emotions can occur at multiple levels of operation, some of which occur consciously and some of which occur automatically. The somatic marker hypothesis also hypothesizes that a defect in emotion and feeling plays an important role in impaired decision making. We would conjecture that this defect represents learned maladaptive behavioral and emotional responses to specific environmental stimuli. There are additional assumptions of the somatic marker hypotheses that also correlate highly with the model of human emotion detailed in our earlier book, *Depathologizing Psychopathology* (2016). Among these are that cognitive processes, regardless of their content, depend on support processes such as attention, working memory, and emotion. In addition, reasoning and decision making depend on the availability of knowledge about situations, actors, options for action and outcomes, and that this knowledge is stored throughout higher-order cortices and some subcortical nuclei.

The important thing to remember about this as far a treatment goes is that these complex stored somatic and cognitive responses and their associated emotional labels can be accessed by triggering any of the associated parts. Thus, a specific situation can trigger the expression of related cognitions and emotional responses, or the somatic response can trigger the expression of the same combination.

Putting Theory into Practice

"Clinical researchers and clinical practitioners share a goal of increasing the integration of research and clinical practice, which is reflected in an evidence-based practice (EBP) approach to psychology. The EBP framework involves the integration of research findings with clinical expertise and client characteristics, values, and preferences, and consequently provides an important foundation for conducting clinically relevant research, as well as empirically based and clinically sensitive practice" (Hershenberg, Drabick, & Vivian, 2012, p. 123). One of the best ways to demonstrate research and practice integration is by the use of case examples. To that end we present the following:

Rhonda

Rhonda was a 38-year-old mother of three who presented in the office with the stated goal of determining whether or not she wished to stay married to her husband of 15 years, George.

Background

Rhonda reported that she and George were high school sweethearts who dated exclusively throughout college and subsequently married. They have three children aged 14, 12, and 8. The oldest and youngest children are girls and the middle child is a boy. Rhonda reported that while they dated George was quite free spirited and fun, and that they enjoyed many shared activities including skiing and traveling. Once they married and the children arrived things began to change. George became increasingly demanding about various aspects of the family functioning. For one thing, George decided about 2 years into the marriage that he would experiment with a vegan lifestyle. The experiment quickly became a passion. George began to demand that the household respect his vegan lifestyle and become vegan entirely. This meant that Rhonda and the children had to be vegan at home even though none of them wished to be. Rhonda offered that it was just easier to comply with the demand as George would fly off into a rage whenever the vegan rule was even mildly breached. The vegan issue was one of several through which George tried to impose his increasingly demanding lifestyle on the other family members. Another area of family disagreement was religion. George had become increasingly devout and wanted the family to attend Sunday services as a family unit as well as participate in other church activities during the week. Lastly, George became increasingly compulsive about cleanliness and appearance. Neither Rhonda nor the children were ever neat enough, or dressed appropriately enough to please George who criticized them constantly for the slightest infraction of his ever escalating set of rules. Rhonda reported that she was always stressed. She described herself as constantly buffering her children from their father's demands and rages. She contended that she would have ended the marriage long before had she not been worried about the children spending time with their father alone.

This scenario led to numerous and escalating confrontations between George and his wife and their older daughter who more openly rebelled against his increasing authoritarianism. Rhonda had to frequently intercede to protect her daughter from George's escalating and violent behavior. Rhonda reported that, due to the incessant criticism she had received from George over the last 10 years, she had becoming increasingly estranged from her husband and could not now identify one thing she actually liked about George. She described interest in sex as nonexistent, although she reported that she would infrequently have relations in order to satisfy his demands in this area. Rhonda reported that George's physical touch repulsed her.

In addition to her questioning her desire to remain in the marriage, Rhonda asked about whether, if he changed, she could ever learn to love George again. This question was precipitated by George recently acknowledging that his behavior was problematic and beginning treatment on his own. Rhonda reported that similar epiphanies had occurred in the past, and while there was some initial improvement, George's old behavioral patterns had always returned.

NCLT practitioners are concerned that their clients understand the model very early on in the therapeutic process. As a result the treatment will start rather quickly. Certainly it is true that the client leaves the first session with a good idea of the process that is about to unfold.

Rhonda's "treatment" began by reformulating her questions in terms of reward valuation. The idea that humans make decisions frequently was explained along with the idea that no one choice was entirely positive or negative. Specifically, divorcing or remaining were choices that had positive and negative attributes to them. Rhonda was asked to consider and innumerate some of these. Protecting the children was a major concern and it was explained that this choice could be argued from either prospective. At the same time, the difference between near term and far term rewards were discussed, and the literature on power dispersement over time was explained. All of this discussion occurred within a context of supporting her through the discussion and having her understand that the role of the therapist was neither to judge nor offer a fool proof decision that did not have consequences. There were either potentially better choices or worse choices, and often times, whether a choice was better or worse would have to await the judgment of history. It was finally explained that choices made currently cannot fully anticipate the future, and that a choice made today that apparently represented the better of two options may, due to circumstances beyond their control, turn out to be the opposite. Cognitive disputational techniques were employed to help her challenge and explore the various rewards and negatives she identified. Rhonda was assigned the homework to list and evaluate as many of the potential rewards and consequences as she could in order to see if a set of options became clearer.

Ronda returned for a second session saying that she had thought through the choices and thought she knew what she wanted to do, but doubted herself and her capacity to make the correct choice. She reported that even as a young child, her mother criticized her ability to make choices and questioned her over all competence. This pattern of self-doubt was exacerbated in her marriage where her husband constantly criticized her behavior. After some discussion using cognitive behavioral techniques to help clarify, it became clear than Rhonda was indeed quite competent at many things. She ran her own successful business and was elected chairperson of her church group on several occasions. She was quite well liked and respected in her community.

Rhonda then asked about the possibility that, if her husband's behavior did indeed change, she would learn to love him again. Both memory reconsolidation theory and learning theory were employed to explain to her what the process might look like. It was explained that she had learned to dislike and distrust her husband over many years composed of many events. Her anxiety and negative arousal states had generalized over the years and would have to be broken down into smaller, controllable events. Each learning circumstance or group of circumstances centering around a theme, vegan food for example, would have to be reprogrammed to more adaptive responses. Each of the circumstances or events was essentially a trigger that could rekindle the memory of her husband as an abusive controlling person at any time and activate the visceral response associated with it. Each trigger would have to be de-potentiated and reattached to a more adaptive response on the part of the husband and a better reaction on the part of the wife. Each time, a challenge to the existing perception, with the added need to address the associated visceral or emotional state, would have to be made. While possible, it would be a massive undertaking and both parties would have to work collaboratively to make it happen. She was asked if she was willing to play her part.

It should be here pointed out that the specific choice Rhonda made was not the crucial therapeutic factor. What mattered was that she was comfortable with her final choice and was able to implement it.

NCLT and Dialectical Behavior Therapy

Dialectical behavior therapy (DBT) places it emphasis on validation, whereby the therapist and the patient work on "accepting" uncomfortable thoughts, feelings, and behaviors rather than struggling with them. Once an identified thought, emotion, or behavior has been validated, the process of change no longer appears difficult, and the process of gradual transformation becomes a reality. The term dialectics refers to the therapist's goal of establishing a balance between acceptance and change and effectively integrating these two fundamental principles of successful therapy. DBT also focuses on the development of coping skills using specific behavioral techniques to combat the disabling symptoms of mental illness (*Dialectical Behavior Therapy*, 2016).

A dialectical behavior therapist (DBT) would perhaps recognize Rhonda at this moment as being in stage two. Rhonda was living a life of depression and desperation. While her behavior was under control, she continued to suffer as a result of past trauma and invalidation. She suspected and inhibited her own emotional responses. In DBT the goal of stage two is to help Rhonda move from a state of quiet desperation to one of full emotional experiencing. NCLT shares in this goal, but adds the goal of how Rhonda got this way, how she is maintaining her behavior (emotional response), and what she could do to change. The careful reader would recognize elements of stage three wherein the challenge for Rhonda is to learn to live: to define life goals, build self-respect, and find peace and happiness. The goal is that the client leads a life of ordinary happiness and unhappiness. NCLT accomplishes this task with a dispassionate analysis of the strengths and weakness of each potential choice. NCLT also adds the understanding of how the pattern of behavior and emotional responding was maintaining, and in fact exacerbating the physiological and self-deprecating responses she had been "taught" and was practicing over the years. Her responses were "depathologized"; how else would one be expected to feel and behave after a lifetime of being berated. NCLT pointed out how this behavioral pattern of backing down was initially adaptive, serving to de-escalate confrontations with her parents, and had become maladaptive when she was no longer in a position of less "power," but continued to react to confrontation as though she was.

At this point in the process Rhonda asked what turned out to be the most pivotal question of the process: "How do I know the choice I make will be the right one" followed quickly with "I don't trust myself to make this choice. So many important people in my life have told me I am incapable, how do I know I am capable?" It is readily apparent that there is no real answer to this question because there is no real way to assess the capability of an individual for each and every situation in which they find themselves. All that could be done was to point out the many areas of competence that she had identified. The therapist concluded that based upon that evidence, Rhonda appeared competent, and as far as the clinician was concerned, if the decision did not work out the way that she wanted it, Ronda had the capability to react and adapt. Rhonda began crying. There are probably a number of ways of looking at this moment including analytic constructs of transference. It was clear from her reaction that the therapist's approval was very important to her. Remember, the approval was of her capability, not one particular choice or another. After a moment Rhonda composed herself. Rhonda left the office saying she knew what she was going to do. She was comfortable in her decision and willing to take a chance on herself.

References

Bechara, A., Damasio, H., & Demasio, A. (2000). Emotion, decision making and the orbitofrontal cortex. *Cerebral Cortex, 10*(3), 295–307. doi:10.1093/cercor/10.3.295.

Beesley, T., Nguyen, K., Pearson, D., & Le Pelley, M. (2015). Uncertainty and predictiveness determine attention to cues during human associative learning. *Quarterly Journal of Experimental Psychology, 68*, 2175–2199. doi:10.1080/17470218.2015.1009919.

Berns, G., Lainson, D., & Lowenstein, G. (2007). Intertemporal choice – Toward an integrative framework. *Trends in Cognitive Neuroscience, 11*(11), 482–488.

Bettman, J., Johnson, E., & Payne, J. (1990). A componential analysis of cognitive effort in choice. *Organizational Behavior and Human Decision Processes, 45*(1), 111–139.

Boddez, Y., Haesen, K., Baeyens, F., & Beckers, T. (2014). Selectivity in associative learning: A cognitive stage framework for blocking and cue competition phenomena. *Frontiers in Psychology, 5*, 1305. doi:10.3389/fpsyg.2014.01305. Retrieved from http://www.ncbi.nlm.nih.gov/pmc/articles/PMC4228836/.

Dialectical behavior therapy. (2016). Retrieved from National Alliance on Mental Illness: https://www2.nami.org/factsheets/DBT_factsheet.pdf

Diederich, A., & Oswald, P. (2014). Sequential sampling model for multiattribute choice alternatives with random attention time and processing order. *Frontiers in Human Neuroscience, 8*, 697. doi:10.3389/fnhum.2014.00697.

Hare, T., Camerer, C., & Rangel, A. (2009). Self-control in decision-making involves modulation of the vmPFC valuation system. *Science, 324*(5927), 646–648. doi:10.1126/science.1168450.

Hershenberg, R., Drabick, D., & Vivian, D. (2012). An opportunity to bridge the gap between clinical research and clinical practice: Implications for clinical training. *Psychotherapy (Chicago, Ill.), 49*(2), 123–134. doi:10.1037/a0027648.

Jack, R., Garrod, O., Yu, H., Caldara, R., & Schyns, P. (2012). Facial expressions of emotion are not culturally universal. *PNAS, 109*(19), 7241–7244. doi:10.1073/pnas.1200155109.

Kruschke, J. (2001). *Cue competition in function learning: Blocking and highlighting.* Retrieved from University of Indiana: http://www.indiana.edu/~kruschke/articles/CueCompFunctLearn. pdf

McClure, S., Laibson, D., Lowenstein, G., & Cohen, J. (2004). Separate neural systems value immediate and delayed monetary rewards. *Science, 306*(5695), 503–507. doi:10.1126/science.1100907.

O'Doherty, J. (2004). Reward representations and reward-related learning in the human. *Current Opinion in Neurobiology, 14*, 768–776. doi:10.1016/j.conb.2004.10.016.

Papez, J. (1937). A proposed mechanism of emotion. *Archives of Neurology and Psychiatry, 38*, 725–743. doi:10.1001/archneurpsyc.1937.0226022006900.

Pichta, M. V., Wolf, R., Lesch, K., Brummer, D., Andreas, C., & Grom, G. (2009). Neural hypo-responsiveness and hyperresponsiveness during immediate and delayed reward processing in adult attention-deficit/hyperactivity disorder. *Biological Psychiatry, 65*(1), 7–14. doi:10.1016/j.biopsych.2008.07.008.

Schultz, W. (2015). Neuronal reward and decision signals: From theories to data. *Physiological Reviews, 95*(3), 853–951. doi:10.1152/physrev.00023.2014.

Wansink, B., & Sobol, J. (2007). Mindless eating the 200 daily food decisions we overlook. *Environment and Behavior, 39*(1), 106–123. doi:10.1177/0013916506295573.

Wasserman, T., & Wasserman, L. (2015). The misnomer of attention-deficit hyperactivity disorder. *Applied Neuropsychology: Child, 4*(2), 116–122. doi:10.1080/21622965.2015.1005487.

Wasserman, T., & Wasserman, L. (2016). *Depathologizing psychopathology.* New York: Springer.

Wittman, M., & Paulus, M. (2008). Decision making, impulsivity and time perception. *Trends in Cognitive Sciences, 12*(1), 7–12. doi:10.1016/j.tics.2007.10.004.

Chapter 6
Memory Reconsolidation and NCLT Practice

What changes in therapy? If therapy works, what changes occur, and how are those changes reflected in everyday life. As might be expected, there are a multiplicity of considerations that have been used to answer this question. Karlsson (2011) reported that psychotherapy outcomes and the mechanisms of change that are related to its effects have traditionally been investigated using psychological and social constructs measured by changes in symptoms, psychological abilities, personality, or social functioning. Oft times these changes are reported quite subjectively. As Kazdin (2007) points out "after decades of psychotherapy research, we cannot provide an evidence-based explanation for how or why even our most well studied interventions produce change, that is, the mechanism(s) through which treatments operate" (p. 1).

This has begun to change, and candidates for the mechanism for change have begun to emerge. For example, as Kazdin (2007) points out, cognitive behavior therapy proposes that changed cognitions cause changed behaviors. More recently, the epigenetic basis of behavior change has been argued (Gottlieb, 2009). NCLT recognizes and incorporates these and other possible mechanisms for behavior change. In addition, NCLT incorporates the research around memory reconsolidation to help explain the deeper, and perhaps more meaningful question which is "What changes in the memory of the individual who has been changed as a result of a therapeutic encounter?" There are several possibilities. For example, when the associations between behaviors and emotions are altered, are the new associations all that are remembered, or does the individual develop and choose a newer, more adaptive set of associations, and merely select them in response to a new stimulus? The literature surrounding memory reconsolidation helps answer this question, and provides important information that informs NCLT practice.

© Springer International Publishing AG 2017
T. Wasserman, L.D. Wasserman, *Neurocognitive Learning Therapy: Theory and Practice*, DOI 10.1007/978-3-319-60849-5_6

Memory Consolidation

To understand memory consolidation, it is necessary to understand how memories get consolidated in the first place. As a reminder, in therapy, we are not attempting to alter the episodic memory. We are attempting to alter the emotional pairing of the memory. Memory consolidation is the processes of first stabilizing and then storing a specific memory trace after it is first acquired. Memory consolidation is usually considered to consist of two specific processes. The first process is called synaptic consolidation, which occurs within the first few hours after learning or encoding. The second process has been termed system consolidation. This occurs when hippocampus-dependent memories become independent of the hippocampus over a period of weeks to years (Maslin, 2010). The process by which this occurs has important implications for NCLT practice.

The process of consolidation is based on a model that uses the concept of long-term potentiation. Long-term potentiation describes a process by which a synapse increases in strength as increasing numbers of signals are transmitted between the two neurons. This strength, or potentiation, is the process by which the synchronous firing of neurons makes those neurons more inclined to fire together in the future. Long-term potentiation occurs when the same group of neurons fire together so often that they become permanently sensitized to each other. As new experiences accumulate, the brain creates more and more connections and pathways, and may "rewire" itself by rerouting connections and rearranging its organization (Maslin, 2010). As this newly established neuronal pathway is utilized over and over again, a relatively permanent pattern is established. Groups of these connected and synchronous pathways between multiple neural structures are called networks. These established networks are more likely to be utilized messages in the future because they represent the path of least resistance for new information to use. This is a major neuronal contribution to the construct of automaticity. The ability of the connection, or synapse, between two neurons to change in strength, and for lasting changes to occur in the efficiency of synaptic transmission, is known as synaptic plasticity or neural plasticity, and it is one of the critical neurochemical foundations of memory and learning.

Clinically speaking, this means that a new client reaching your office will have many clearly established and developed networks that they have developed and rely upon for use when they encounter new information. The important clinical question becomes whether or not these established networks can be changed, and that's where memory reconsolidation comes in.

Memory Reconsolidation

Memory reconsolidation is the process of previously consolidated memories being recalled, and then actively consolidated all over again, in order to maintain, strengthen, and modify memories that are already stored in the long-term memory.

The very act of reconsolidation though, may change the initial memory. As a particular memory trace is reactivated, the strengths of the neural connections may change. Importantly for NCLT practice, the memory may become associated with new emotional or environmental conditions or subsequently acquired knowledge. At this stage, expectations, rather than actual events, may become incorporated into the memory.

Recent research has demonstrated that psychotherapies can be integrated via their common ability to trigger the neurobiological mechanism of memory reconsolidation in such a way as to lead to deconsolidation of a previously learned emotional response and the reconsolidation of a more adaptive response (Ecker, Ticic, & Hulley, 2013). It is important to remember that the term "reconsolidation" has two slightly different meanings. Reconsolidation describes the relocking of synapses in the final step of the natural process of synaptic unlocking and relocking that is part of the regular memory process. It also refers to the overall process of unlocking, revising, and then relocking the synapses encoding a specific memory. It is this second operation that is vitally important in therapy. "It is now clear that the consolidation of emotional memory is not, as had been believed for a century, a one-time, final process, and that emotional learning is not indelible. Rather, neural circuits encoding an emotional learning can be returned to a de-consolidated state, allowing erasure by new learnings before a relocking (reconsolidation) takes place. Counteracting and regulating unwanted acquired responses is not the best one can do because emotional learnings can be dissolved, not just suppressed" (Ecker et al., 2013, p. 84). In other words, they can be changed permanently. It is also important to note that after a learned emotional response has been eliminated through the reconsolidation process, the individual will still remember the experiences in which the response was acquired, the stimuli to which it was originally associated as well as the fact of having had the response in the first place. It is that the emotional response itself is no longer re-evoked by remembering those experiences.

More important additional research demonstrated that memory reactivation alone was not sufficient for unlocking the synapses encoding a target learning (Pedreira, Pérez-Cuesta, & Maldonado, 2004) thereby triggering deconsolidation of the original memory and reconsolidation of the new desired memory. In order for deconsolidation to occur, a critical additional experience must take place while the memory is still reactivated. This second experience consists of perceptions that significantly mismatch from what the reactivated target memory expects and predicts about how the world functions. Additional research suggests that behavioral interference paradigms have been the most successful at demonstrating evidence for reconsolidation in humans (Schiller & Phellps, 2011). This clearly implies that behavioral practice that incorporates the new adaptive cognitive coping statement must be incorporated into every therapy session.

This deconsolidation, and then reconsolidation in a different form, is triggered by a violation of expectation (prediction) based upon prior learning. This violation can be qualitative (the outcome not occurring at all), or quantitative (the magnitude of the outcome not being fully predicted). Lee (2009) proposed that "the existence of a prediction error signal (from some brain region)] might be a crucial pre-requisite for reconsolidation to be triggered" (p. 419).

It is also clear the reconsolidation of memory affects different memory systems differently. For amygdala-dependent expressions of fear learning and emotion-based learning, information during reconsolidation appears to rewrite or overwrite the original fear memory (Schiller et al., 2010). When examining hippocampal-dependent episodic memory, the primary content of this original episodic memory appears to be relatively intact following interference during reconsolidation, but the memory is now confused or merged with the interfering information. This latter finding demonstrates why the experiences in therapy must be paired with physiologically, emotionally based arousal in order for the treatment to work to its maximum effectiveness.

Finally, memorized behavioral skills presenting an interfering motor skill during reconsolidation result in impaired expression of the original skill memory, but there still evidence that it exists, although in a less automatic state.

The Linkages Between All Aspects of Memory

Although the above may suggest that the memory components are independent of each other, there is substantial research to suggest that emotional responses, autobiographical memories, episodic and semantic structures derived from them are firmly interconnected (Lane, Ryan, Nadel, & Greenberg, 2015). "Together they form an integrated memory structure that can be accessed by many cues and emotional responses including action tendencies and behaviors expressive of emotion, perceptual details associated with the event (s), and the derived principles, rules, and schemas used to interpret novel situations. All of those elements have the ability to activate the memory structure, and importantly, once activated, any one of the components has the potential to update other components of the structure via reconsolidation. Emotional responding is not separate from the event memories that occurred when that response was first experienced. Nor are semantic structures accessed without reinstating personally relevant information, and, particularly under circumstances where the memory was strongly reconsolidated, the specific memories that add unique information to that structure" (p. 14).

How Is Memory Reconsolidation Used in Therapy?

Prior to beginning deconsolidation Ecker, Ticic, and Hulley (2013, p. 91) identify a preparatory process to be used clinically. This process consists of three steps:

1. *Symptom identification.* Actively clarify with the client what to regard as the presenting symptom(s) including the specific behaviors, somatics, emotions, and/or thoughts that the client wants to eliminate. Identify when they happen, that is, the cues, associated stimuli, and contexts that evoke or intensify them.

2. *Retrieval of target learning.* Retrieve into explicit awareness, as a visceral emotional experience, the details of the emotional learning or schema underlying and driving the presenting symptom.

3. *Identification of disconfirming knowledge.* "Identify a vivid experience (past or present) that can serve as living knowledge that is fundamentally incompatible with the model of reality in the target emotional learning retrieved in step B, such that both cannot possibly be true. The disconfirming material may or may not be appealing to the client as being more 'positive' or preferred; what matters is that it be mutually exclusive, ontologically, with the target learning. It may be already part of the client's personal knowledge or may be created by a new experience" (p. 91)

Ecker et al. (2013) then go on to provide an outline of the behavioral process of transformational change of an existing and likely maladaptive emotional learning/ behavioral pairing that correspond to the way that the brain processes information that we have outlined earlier. They identify three essential steps:

1. *Reactivate the automated emotional response to the stimuli, cue, or trigger.* The therapist accomplishes this by re-triggering/re-evoking the target knowledge by presenting salient cues or contexts from the original learning.

2. *Create a mismatch that unlocks/deconsolidates the original automated cue response pair.* While the reactivation is occurring, create an experience that is significantly at variance with the target learning's model and predicted expectations of how the world functions. This step unlocks synapses and renders memory circuits labile (neural plasticity), and therefore susceptible to being updated by new learning.

3. *Erase or revise via new learning.* Create a new learning experience that contradicts (for erasing) or supplements (for revising) the labile target knowledge. This new learning experience may be the same as, or different from the experience used for mismatch in step 2; if it is the same, step 3 consists of repetitions of step 2. As the window of neural plasticity is hypothesized to be somewhat short (5 h or so), it is necessary for the disconfirming pairings to be practiced as part of the session.

NCLT and Memory Reconsolidation

NCLT practice incorporates this body of knowledge into its core operational procedures. In line with Ecker et al. (2013) we recognize that "new learning always creates new neural circuits, but transformational change occurs only when new learning radically unlearns, unwires and replaces an existing learning, rather than merely forming alongside existing learning and competitively regulating it. The use of new learning to erase an existing, unwanted learning is precisely what the therapeutic reconsolidation process achieves. It consists of steps that guide therapy, yet allow an extremely broad range of techniques to be used for guiding the key experiences, so a therapist's individual style of working continues to have great scope of expression" (p. 95). This is a crucial point for NCLT practice. NCLT makes use of this knowledge and, as a result, permits the incorporation of many types of therapeutic encounters and systems. It does not matter what system you use as long as it is used for the right purpose and in the right way. That is as long as it is used to disconfirm prior knowledge so that different conclusions and associations can be reached.

How Do You Know That the New Learning Has Been Consolidated? (How Do You Know When You Have Been Successful?)

There is currently no way to map individual connectomes and thus no way to physiologically determine whether memory has been reconfigured. There are characteristics of learning that we can observe that will provide the therapist with important clues about memory configuration (Ecker et al., 2013). These are the following:

1. *Non-reactivation*: A specific emotional reaction that was initially produced in response to a stimulus suddenly and consistently can no longer be reactivated by cues and triggers that formerly did so.
2. *Symptom cessation*: Symptoms of behavior, emotion, physiological responses or thought that were expressions of, and associated with, the emotional reaction in question also disappear permanently.
3. *Effortless permanence*: The previously maladaptive emotional and behavioral responses do not recur even when counteractive or preventative measures of any kind are terminated.

As we have learned above these assessments most clearly pertain to emotionally based memories.

Generalization Is Essential

The deconsolidation/reconsolidation of a new emotional and behavioral pairing is initially quite targeted and specific. Research has demonstrated that when a deconsolidated memory is unlearned and essentially reconstituted as a more adaptive response, the reconstitution is limited to precisely the reactivated target learning, without impairing other closely linked emotional learnings that have not been directly reactivated (Schiller et al., 2010). Clinically this clearly implies that in order to become a fully automated response to many types of stressful situations, these new pairings must be practiced in response to many different cues that in the past had evoked the undesirable emotional response. As we have indicated elsewhere, these practice sessions must be planned and targeted, and involve a realistic situation.

The Glass Shattering: An Example

Violet had been in therapy for a considerable period of time. The subject of her poor self-image permeated our sessions and remained rather resistant to modification. The only area Violet felt good about herself in was her capacity as a teacher. Violet had been deprecated by her parents on a regular basis, having been told repeatedly as a young girl that she was not pretty, too fat, etc. through therapy Violet had come to understand that her pervasive anxiety was the result of her repeated exposure to negative comments. At one point in our therapeutic process this topic of self-deprecation came up again. Finally, Violet was able to articulate her core belief. Violet believed that the abuse was in fact her own fault. As proof of her deprecation being her own fault Violet offered "Well, wasn't it? My mother was beautiful." Violet was then to consider the implication of her statement and was asked "So, only beautiful people have worth. I guess we should just terminate anyone who is not attractive. Whose children should we start with?" Violet literally stopped all movement, and then described the impact of this as "a glass shattering."

In terms of memory reconsolidation, we can understand this moment in the following way; From a clinical perspective, the automated emotional response was triggered and a concept significantly at variance with the targeted learning was introduced; Violet was very proud of her teaching skills and the accomplishments of her students. The idea of establishing their worth based upon their attractiveness was incompatible with her values. From a neurobiological perspective, the synapses were labile and available for updating by the new learning. It is the moment when the old automated response was challenged and could no longer be held without question. It was when the networked response was available for modification. In other words, it was the successful process of therapy.

In this instance it is noteworthy that Violet was not introduced to a completely new value. Violet would always have been horrified to think that she would not value one of her students based upon their physical appearance. She had never applied the same standard to herself. When the two standards were juxtaposed, Violet could not maintain both. One of them had to go. Violet, being essentially sound, chose the one representing a higher standard; All people have worth, regardless of their physical appearance.

Therapeutic Practice and the NCLT System

An extremely broad range of techniques can be used to carry out the process of memory reconsolidation. That is why the creativity and individual style of the therapist continue to have great scope of expression. As the research demonstrates, many different types of therapeutic interventions can produce memory reconsolidation, and as of yet, no single school can claim hegemony as to whom does it better (Ecker, Ticic, & Hulley, 2012). Indeed, there are other therapeutic models such as the emotional coherence framework (Ecker et al., 2012) that utilize this basic fact of memory change as the basis for their systems of change. What sets NCLT apart is that NCLT specifically combines the understanding of memory reconsolidation with the basic understanding of how the brain processes the very information that it uses to reconsolidate memory. Other therapeutic systems speculate how the various treatments impact the emotional processes of the individual. NCLT postulates how these interventions are actually used by the brain. Combining these two bodies of research provides the practitioner with a powerful set of tools with which to effect therapeutic change.

In fact, a number of existing systems of psychotherapy have been identified in the research as effective and compatible with carrying out the memory reconsolidation process. These include EMDR (Solomon & Shapiro, 2008), coherence therapy (Ecker et al., 2013), behavioral and cognitive behavior therapy (Lane et al., 2015), psychodynamic therapy models (Lane et al., 2015), and Gestalt therapeutic paradigms (Kandel, 2001). As in the coherence therapy framework all of these therapeutic systems can be used within an NCLT framework as long as the appropriate procedures are utilized to insure the memory reconsolidation process takes place.

References

Ecker, B., Ticic, R., & Hulley, L. (2012). *Unlocking the emotional brain eliminating symptoms at their roots using memory reconsolidation*. East Sussex, UK: Routledge.

Ecker, B., Ticic, R., & Hulley, L. (2013). A primer on memory reconsolidation and its psychotherapeutic use as a core process of profound change. *Neuropsychotherapist, 1*, 82–99. doi:10.12744/tnpt(1)082-099.

Gottlieb, G. (2009). *Individual development and evolution*. Marwah, NJ: Lawrence Erlbaum and Associates.

Kandel, E. (2001). The molecular biology of memory storage: A dialogue between genes and synapses. *Science, 294*(5544), 1030–1038. doi:10.1126/science.1067020.

Karlsson, H. (2011, August). How psychotherapy changes the brain. *Psychiatric Times*, p. 1.

Kazdin, A. (2007). Mediators and mechanisms of change in psychotherapy research. *Annual Review of Clinical Psychology, 3*, 1–27. doi:10.1146/annurev.clinpsy.3.022806.091432.

Lane, R., Ryan, L., Nadel, L., & Greenberg, L. (2015). Memory reconsolidation, emotional arousal, and the process of change in psychotherapy: New insights from brain science. *Behavioral and Brain Sciences, e1*, 1–64. doi:10.1017/S0140525X14000041.

Lee, L. (2009). Reconsolidation: Maintaining memory relevance. *Trends in Neuroscience, 32*, 413–420. doi:10.1016/j.tins.2009.05.002.

Maslin, L. (2010). *Memory consolidation*. Retrieved from The Human Memroy: http://www.human-memory.net/processes_consolidation.html

Pedreira, M., Pérez-Cuesta, L., & Maldonado, H. (2004). Mismatch between what is expected and what actually occurs triggers memory reconsolidation or extinction. *Learning & Memory, 11*, 579–585. doi:10.1101/lm.76904.

Schiller, D., Monfils, M.-H., Raio, C. M., Johnson, D. C., LeDoux, J. E., & Phelps, E. A. (2010). Preventing the return of fear in humans using reconsolidation update mechanisms. *Nature, 463*, 49–53. doi:10.1038/nature08637.

Schiller, D., & Phellps, E. (2011). Does reconsolidation occur in humans? *Frontiers in Behavioral Neuroscience, 5*(24). doi:10.3389/fnbeh.2011.00024. Retrieved from http://journal.frontiersin.org/article/10.3389/fnbeh.2011.00024/full.

Solomon, R., & Shapiro, F. (2008). EMDR and the adaptive information processing model. *Journal of EMDR Practice and Research, 2*(4), 315–325.

Chapter 7
Automaticity

Why Automaticity?

As we indicated earlier, automaticity is a key construct and consideration in NCLT practice. Automaticity is defined herein as the desired outcome of learning. Automaticity has also been termed instrumental learning. Braunlich & Seger (2013) divide instrumental learning into two types, goal directed and habitual. They point out that this habitual behavior (automatic) is elicited by environmental stimuli, and develops to a point that it occurs without conscious consideration of outcome. It is behavior that has become so practiced; it is automatically engaged and expressed. Goal-directed behavior assesses the contingencies between our behavior and potential outcomes. In this volume we have described that assessment process as based on the construct of reward recognition and have identified neural networks dedicated to that process. Once the reward value of a solution has been established and selected, it occurs almost every time that the stimuli that evoked it is encountered. Once that behavior is sufficiently practiced, it enters a state of automaticity.

Automaticity is not limited to observable motor behaviors. It refers to the learning of behaviors which require attention, focus, and working memory. Koziol and Budding (2009) discuss how we require a system which will allow us to "know what to do". This automatic system is designed to handle the well-rehearsed or routine responses and thoughts, and then extend to the development of a problem solving system for unfamiliar or novel circumstances. Automization therefore refers to behaviors and the plans, cognitions, and responses that are related to those behaviors.

The understanding of automaticity is essential to both the NCLT conceptualization of the development of mental dysfunction and the creation of a system of intervention required to address it.

© Springer International Publishing AG 2017
T. Wasserman, L.D. Wasserman, *Neurocognitive Learning Therapy: Theory and Practice*, DOI 10.1007/978-3-319-60849-5_7

The Role of Automaticity in NCLT Practice

NCLT theory posits that much of what is currently defined as mental disorder actually reflects the development of maladaptive behaviors, thoughts, feelings, and/or visceral responses which have become automatic. These maladaptive response tendencies are then inappropriately applied or selected for use in response to specific stimuli. By the process of response generalization these habitual or automatic maladaptive response tendencies are then extended onto novel situations, thereby developing into generalized response tendencies labeled as disorders. NCLT theory also posits that the individual recognizes the trend of strengthening the automaticity of the generalized and interconnected response tendency that results in outcomes which by themselves cause emotional and mental distress because of recognition of the misapplication and poor section bias. In simpler terms, this means that clients become increasingly distressed because they keep engaging in responses that they know are not adaptive (Chan & Mac, 2015). Directly stated, this is the therapeutic answer that should be used when the client asked the oft repeated refrain "Why do I keep doing this?"

The Use of Automization in Therapy

NCLT is not the only therapeutic approach to incorporate the understanding of automization as part of treatment paradigms. Cognitive behavioral approaches also incorporate an understanding of concepts such as patient bias as automated cognitive responses (McNally, 1995). Self-instructional training, initially used with hyperactive children to change maladaptive thinking processes, stress inoculation training used to alter conceptualizations about perceive stressful stimuli, and coping skills training used to confront stressful situations all rely heavily on automating adaptive responses to replace maladaptive ones (Meichenbaum, 1977). Finally, automatic response behavior has been considered to be an important etiological consideration in the mindfulness strategies used in the cognitive behavioral treatment of anxiety disorders (Carmody, 2015) and depression (Lang, 2013). Like these other techniques, NCLT recognizes that adaptive and maladaptive behaviors occur at the automatic level, and that much of human behavior, good and bad, occurs at the automatic level because the architecture and capacity of the human brain require that heavily practiced routines be conducted effortlessly and efficiently.

Automaticity, Learning Theory, and Therapy

What exactly then is automaticity in a learning theory context and how might it be used in therapy? NCLT makes use of the following definition: an automatic process is one that once initiated (regardless of whether it was initiated intentionally or unintentionally), runs to completion with no requirement for conscious guidance, cognitive effort, or monitoring (Moors & De Houwer, 2006). Because it runs in the background, there is no impact on cognitive load and no effect on cognitive demand.

In addition, in agreement with Bargh (1992), therapeutic intervention based on vertical brain-based learning theory is conducted on the idea that all automatic processes are conditional. This means that they are all dependent on certain preconditions. For example, autonomous processes require the presence of a triggering stimulus, awareness and recognition of a stimulus, the intention for the process to take place, the expenditure of attentional resources, and the salience of the stimulus. Automatic processes will vary with regard as to the specific subset of preconditions they require. Because of their role as triggering agents, the identification of these preconditions becomes an important element of the therapeutic process.

Triggers and Their Role in Therapy

We can now recognize that most therapy processes emphasize the identification of these environmental triggers and the automatized response to them. This is usually the first step in many therapeutic processes, and certainly among the first thing one would do in an NCLT session. This is because most every therapeutic model understands that the sequence of reaction starts with the identification of a trigger. For example, cognitive behavior therapy starts with the identification of an external trigger (an event, a situation, a series of circumstances) or internal trigger (a feeling, a physical sensation, anticipatory thoughts about a projected situation) that produces a response characterized as a series of thoughts or graphic responses (cognitive response). Therapy, in a cognitive behavioral model, is about identifying the triggers and changing the cognitive descriptions of them in the hopes of getting the individual to select a more adaptive response.

While different therapy approaches vary on how to identify these triggers and how to reprogram them, all are in agreement that the primary task of therapy is the same; the reprogramming of maladaptive, automatized responses to adaptive ones. While it may be true that in certain instances a client may be upset over a patterned response in which they engage, it is usually the case that the client is befuddled about why they selected that response in the first place. For example, most people with Obsessive Compulsive Disorder know that their obsessions and compulsions are foolish, yet they do them anyway (Greybiel & Rausch, 2000). In fact, the responses can range from somewhat foolish to fully hampering. Still, they engage in these maladaptive responses. People are usually looking for the why of the matter, seeking to offer a reasonable explanation for the behaviors or obsessions, and often pick the most obvious explanation, regardless of whether the explanation was in fact a factor or not. There are, to be sure, different ways of describing the process and the outcome. Whether you are talking about cognitive change or self-actualization, you are describing a new set of adaptive responses to environmental exigencies. The label you use to describe your success may be different, but the results are comprised of related action tendencies on the part of the person.

Automatization and the Unconscious

We have discussed the relationship of the two constructs of automatization and the unconscious elsewhere (Wasserman & Wasserman, 2016); however, it is important to point out here that NCLT does not rule out understanding that certain actions and decisions are arrived at by using processes that operate below the threshold of conscious awareness. The difference between NCLT and classically termed psychodynamic models is that NCLT posits that the below awareness triggers are the result of exposure and practice as opposed to drives and desires specific to the realm of the unconscious. NCLT practice would strive to make the rules and specific triggers governing these highly automatic routines knowable, and therefore modifiable. This is quite different from psychodynamic models that discuss the operation of unconscious drives.

NCLT does not take issue with the idea of unconscious cognitive processes, but instead embraces the idea that these processes are critically important to the development and maintenance of emotional states. Research has demonstrated that nonconscious processes produced the same outcomes as their conscious counterparts, across a variety of behavioral domains (Bargh, Gollwitzer, Lee-Chai, Barndollar, & Troetschel, 2001). In addition, nonconsciously primed concepts can exert significant directive influences over behavior (Aarts & Dijksterhuis, 2003), suggesting that an important source of the impulses from which human action and response emanates, may be automatic environmental priming effects.

Questions About the Role of Automatization in Therapy

The scientific questions pertaining to therapy that can be derived from a recognition that automaticity is perhaps the most important process to be managed during the therapeutic process are direct ones:

Is there an efficient way to perform this process of de-automating maladaptive responses and re-automating adaptive ones?

If there are several ways to achieve this end is one more efficient than the others?

Is efficiency the goal or is one process better at producing greater knowledge acquisition at the expense of time?

Is there a process that produces lasting change that generalized to other related aspects of behavior?

While these are all questions that deserve answers based on scientific inquiry, we do not seek to answer them, or answer any of them as regards every therapeutic system. Rather, we will answer them from an NCLT perspective because we have every confidence that the process we describe has been validated by the research we have outlined to produce permanent and generalized automated adaptive cognitive and behavioral responses. What we will clarify is what is now known, and that is that the brain processes information in a predictable fashion, both consciously and unconsciously. The question we seek to answer is whether there is a particular form of therapeutic information provision that makes maximum effectiveness of the information based upon the manner that is consistent with how the brain is going to process it. The answer to that is that there are specific principles of brain-based learning that are directly applicable to the therapeutic process, and that these should be incorporated into standard therapeutic practice. These principles are incorporated into NCLT.

NCLT Answers to Questions Concerning the Role of Automaticity

For NCLT the role of automaticity in the therapy process emphasizes that automatized maladaptive behavioral and cognitive processes be first made available to working memory and attention and then systematically altered with the resulting adaptive processes re-automatized. This procedure occurs in several discrete stages for each problem identified:

1. The recognition by the client that there are automatic processes driving the current problematic behavior and thinking.
2. The recognition by the client that these processes are the result of learning.
3. The identification of specific triggers.
4. The identification and specification of the rules governing specific processes.
5. Memory reconsolidation work designed to challenge the existing rule structure and establish a more adaptive set of responses.
6. Creation of a new adaptive process.
7. Practice of the new rule process in the therapeutic setting.
8. Practice of the new process in the environment to encourage generalization.

Automaticity, Learning, and Disease

For NCLT, most maladaptive responses and the reformulated adaptive ones are learned. They do not come preprogrammed at the factory. They represent the interaction of core temperamental characteristics (Chess & Thomas, 1967) and regulatory efficiency with environmental experiences. The fact that they are learned (or shaped through an experiential process) can be unlearned and adaptively relearned means, that for the most, part we are not dealing with a disease process. A disease can be defined in several ways such as "any impairment of normal physiological function affecting all or part of an organism, esp. a specific pathological change caused by infection, stress, etc., producing characteristic symptoms; illness or sickness in general" (Reverso, 2014) or pathology (Perry et al., 2008). Either definition implies that there is some disruption of the normal.

Small world hub models, and the related construct of automaticity, imply that the network of connectionist hubs is unique to each human being. Some may be adaptive and some maladaptive, but the vast majority of these networks are based on the systems responses to the environmental stimuli it encounters. They are created by learning and are the result of that learning. In recognizing that, it becomes important to consider that learning and educational processes and principles should be utilized when trying to alter these processes.

A Note About Journaling

We frequently encounter patients who have been previously been in therapy. It is not uncommon for some of them to very proudly offer that, as they had been instructed by their prior therapist, they have gone back to journaling. We always want to reinforce a client for initiative and effort. In keeping with this, we might offer some confirmation of their efforts. However, NCLT does not endorse nondirected journaling. Remember, learning is achieved through practice. It is not helpful to our clients to be practicing self-defeating and/or negative thought processes through their writing. Repeating some variant of "I feel so depressed" is not helpful to the therapeutic process as it releases a cascade of neurophysiological processes to neurophysiologically reinforce (make automatic) that emotional state. Consequently, the practice of negative statements and emotions would only serve to reinforce their automaticity. Rather, journaling toward problem solving of their emotional states and dilemmas, keeping in line with the above outlined stages, is encouraged.

Automaticity and Small World Hub Algorithms

As regards automatization, therapy process based on a small world hub model of brain organization would utilize an algorithm strengthening model (Anderson, 1996) that proposes one single learning mechanism to account for automatization of all routines. An algorithm is a mathematically understandable and expressible cognitive process. Automaticity is largely about efficiency and the algorithmic models developed to describe it are called algorithmic efficiency theories.

Algorithmic Efficiency Theories

The central theme of algorithm efficiency theories is that practice improves the efficiency (speed and fluidity) of the underlying algorithmic processes that compute interpretations of task stimuli (Rawson, 2010). In an algorithm strengthening model, consistent practice is essential for the development of automaticity. Improvement in terms of efficiency requires algorithms to remain consistent with practice, even though aspects of the data they are practiced upon may change. For example, when a student is learning addition, the algorithm (process) is the same wither the number involved is a 2, or a 3, or a 45 (Carlson & Lundy, 1992). This principle would suggest that sound therapeutic process would involve systematic and direct practice of the new skill (belief). This practice should include behaviors that devolve from the expression of the belief. For example, if a person comes to believe that Yoga is beneficial, it is not sufficient to merely practice the statement that yoga is beneficial, but it is usually required to practice the behaviors (doing the Yoga) that devolve from incorporating that belief. This principle would also imply that the clearer the connection is between the belief and the practice, the more efficiently it will be learned.

The Act Principle

There are some additional aspects of these algorithmic models that have implications for NCLT therapeutic practice. One of them is called the algorithm (processing) strengthening (Adaptive Control of Thought or ACT) principle. This principle states that the same algorithms responsible for the initial, nonautomatic stage of performance are also responsible for the skilled, automatic stage of performance. In the latter stage, these algorithms are executed faster and more efficiently with increasingly less conscious allocation of working memory and control required. Hence, automatic and nonautomatic algorithms differ only with regard to the features (such as speed and efficiency) they possess (Rawson, 2010). This clearly implies that awareness and knowledge of how these algorithms operate both on a conceptual and neurophysiological level is essential for the therapist when designating intervention strategies, because there is only one set of algorithms that will control the sequence of the behavior during both the acquisition stage and the demonstration stage. It also implies that a planned and purposeful creation of the algorithms that has predictable outcomes would be preferable to a haphazard one.

Vertical Brain Implications of Automaticity

Vertical brain-based therapy principles also emphasize the role of attention in automaticity (Koziol & Budding, 2009). Attending to a stimulus is necessary to encode it initially into working memory, or to retrieve from long-term memory. Attention is a form of selection wherein the individual allocates working memory to a specific stimulus (Shell et al., 2010). When a stimulus is either encoded or retrieved, all information that was associated with it during a former presentation are attended to as well. Both storage and retrieval are improved each time attention is focused on the stimulus. Retrieval is done with less effort each time. In addition, as retrieval efficiency is improved, stronger retrieval cues are created, and automatic retrieval becomes ever more likely.

Consider a client for a moment. Now consider a reconceptualization of their presenting symptoms. Consider the implications for multiple emotional and behavioral response patterns you have witnessed occurring in your clients. Consider the strength of the neurophysiological connections—the number of times, the number of years they have practiced this response—of your client's responses. Now, consider the new way you would frame this for your client.

Automatization produces a shift in attention (rather than a reduction), with attention being allocated to higher levels of organization. When components of a skill become automatic with practice, attention is shifted from them to higher-level aspects of the skill concerned with the integration of complex skills (Logan, 1992). The implications for therapy become clear. Older maladaptive behaviors are expressed automatically in response to a variety of highly integrated stimuli. These stimuli must be re-paired with adaptive routines which are at first highly cognitive, unpracticed, and rough. These new routines, which require considerable cognitive effort, are difficult to learn, and at first, highly specific to the situation in which they are learned. Successful therapy encourages the practice of these new adaptive routines until they become widely responsive to a variety of cues, automatic, practiced, and efficient. Automaticity would reciprocally improve the selection process as well. For example, successful treatment for a person with a negative outlook, or depression, would involve having a person spontaneously identify the potential in a difficult situation, as opposed to seeing only the dangers.

References

Aarts, H., & Dijksterhuis, A. (2003). The silence of the library: Environment, situational norm, and social behavior. *Journal of Personality and Social Psychology, 84*, 18–28.

Anderson, J. R. (1996). ACT: A simple theory of complex cognition. *American Psychologist, 51*, 355–365.

Bargh, J. A. (1992). The ecology of automaticity: Toward establishing the conditions needed to produce automatic processing effects. *American Journal of Psychology, 105*, 181–199.

Bargh, J. A., Gollwitzer, P., Lee-Chai, A., Barndollar, K., & Troetschel, R. (2001). The automated will: Nonconscious activation and pursuit of behavioral goals. *Journal of Personality and Social Psychology, 81*, 1014–1027.

Braunlich, K., & Seger, C. (2013). The basal ganglia. *WIREs Cognitive Science, 4*, 135–148. doi:10.1002/wcs.1217.

Carlson, R. A., & Lundy, D. H. (1992). Consistency and restructuring in cognitive procedural sequences. *Journal of Experimental Psychology: Learning, Memory, and Cognition, 18*, 127–141.

Carmody, J. (2015). Mindfulness as a general ingredient of successful psychotherapy. In B. Ostafin, M. Robinson, & B. Meier (Eds.), *Handbook of mindfulness and self-regulation* (pp. 235–248). New York: Springer.

Chan, K., & Mac, W. (2015). Habitual self-stigma: The contributory role of maladaptive coping with self-stigmatizing thoughts. *European Psychiatry, 30*(Suppl 1), 739.

Chess, S., & Thomas, A. B. (1967). Behavior problems revisited: Findings of an anterospective study. *Journal of the American Academy of Child Psychiatry, 6*(2), 321–331.

Greybiel, A., & Rausch, S. (2000). Toward a neurobiology of obsessive-compulsive disorder. *Neuron, 28*(2), 343–347.

Koziol, K., & Budding, D. (2009). *Subcortical structures and cognition*. New York: Springer.

Lang, A. (2013). What mindfullness brings to psychotherapy for anxiety and depression. *Depression and Anxiety, 30*(5), 409–412. doi:10.1002/da.22081.

Logan, G. D. (1992). Attention and preattention in theories of automaticity. *American Journal of Psychology, 105*, 317–339.

McNally, R. (1995). Automaticity and the anxiety disorders. *Behaviour Research and Therapy, 33*(7), 747–754.

Meichenbaum, D. (1977). Cognitive behaviour modification. *Scandinavian Journal of Behaviour Therapy, 6*(4), 185–192.

Moors, A., & De Houwer, J. (2006). Automaticity: A theoretical and conceptual analysis. *Psychological Bulletin, 132*(2), 297–326. doi:10.1037/0033-2909.132.2.297.

Perry, G., Castellani, R., Moreira, P., Lee, H., Zhu, X., & Smith, M. (2008). Pathology's new role: Defining disease process and protective responses. *International Journal of Clinical and Experimental Pathology, 1*(1), 1–4.

Rawson, K. (2010). Defining and investigating automaticity in reading. In B. Ross (Ed.), *The psychology of learning and motivation* (pp. 185–230). Burlington, NJ: Elsevier.

Reverso. (2014). *Disease process definition*. Retrieved from Reverso: http://dictionary.reverso.net/english-definition/disease%20process

Shell, D., Brooks, D., Trainin, G., Wilson, K., Kauffman, D., & Herr, L. (2010). *The unified learning model how motivational, cognitive, and neurobiological sciences inform best teaching practices*. New York: Springer.

Wasserman, T., & Wasserman, L. (2016). *Depathologizing psychopathology*. New York: Springer.

Part II
The Clinical Practice of Neurocognitive Learning Therapy

Chapter 8
How to Be an NCLT Therapist

NCLT Is Not Eclecticism

Perhaps one of the most difficult things to describe is how your practice behavior defines you as an NCLT therapist. If, as we have said, you can utilize a number of therapeutic intervention models as part of NCLT practice, what is it that you do or believe that sets you apart from practitioners of other models?

For example, it could be conceivable that a cognitive behavior therapist or a non-directive therapist, who describes themselves an eclectic when it comes to using different techniques for different problems, could argue that they were following the NCLT model. In fact, a short answer to the above question is that one could describe oneself in that manner and still do many of the things we have spoken about as characterizing NCLT. Even better, you can describe yourself as eclectic and avoid the discussion altogether. However, these and similar descriptions miss the heart and soul of what constitutes NCLT practice. Much of what it spoken about when individuals describe what kind of practitioner they are have to do with the type of intervention they conduct. Cognitive behavior therapists modify maladaptive cognitions, and behavior therapists modify maladaptive behaviors. Neither of these two disciplines can point to a current, empirically valid model of mental health development as the underpinning for issues of mental health. They continue to exist because they are effective at altering aspects of behavior or cognition that are associated with disorders of mental health and to use these models therapeutically, it is not required to hold with a model of mental health development at all. You simply change maladaptive activities to adaptive ones. Perhaps psychoanalysis is the exception to this rule in that it is based on a model of resolution of early developing conflict. Psychoanalytic theory, albeit developed by a neurologist, and quit sophisticated for its time, has had difficulty integrating itself with current neurobiological psychiatry. In fact, the models are frequently at odds with one another (Robbins, 1992). In addition, concepts such as anxiety being caused when parts of the unconscious mind,

© Springer International Publishing AG 2017
T. Wasserman, L.D. Wasserman, *Neurocognitive Learning Therapy: Theory and Practice*, DOI 10.1007/978-3-319-60849-5_8

specifically the id and superego, are in constant conflict with the conscious part of the mind, represented by the ego, find very little research support.

So when you say you are an NCLT therapist what are you communicating to your clients and fellow practitioners?

NCLT Practice Is About the Model

The first and foremost thing that characterizes the work of an NCLT therapist is that all intervention is derived from understanding a very specific model concerning the development of mental health in general and problems of mental health in specific. This is an important distinction in that the NCLT model can be used to describe the development of adaptive behavior or account for the development of a mentally healthy individual. It is as much as discussion of mental health as it is a discussion of mental disorder. As we have seen, this model is life course in nature and in many instances does not require the discussion of disease. As we have seen, NCLT is built around three foundational/principle areas of research: learning theory, probabilistic reward valuation, and memory reconsolidation. These are at the core of NCLT modeling and you cannot claim to be an NCLT practitioner unless these principles are part of your everyday practice. In this chapter we will look at other elements of therapeutic practice that help delineate an individual as an NCLT practitioner.

A Word About Disease and Disorder

The astute reader has probably noticed by now that the term "disease" is rarely used in NCLT practice. To a lesser extent, the same can be said about the word disorder. Disease is defined in a couple of different ways. The Merriam Webster dictionary defines the term as follows: "a condition of the living animal or plant body or of one of its parts that impairs normal functioning and is typically manifested by distinguishing signs and symptoms" or an "illness that affects a person, animal, or plant: a condition that prevents the body or mind from working normally" (Merriam Webster, 2016) or this "disordered or incorrectly functioning organ, part, structure, or system of the body resulting from the effect of genetic or developmental errors, infection, poisons, nutritional deficiency or imbalance, toxicity, or unfavorable environmental factors; illness, sickness," or finally this: "any impairment of normal physiological function affecting all or part of an organism, esp. a specific pathological change caused by infection, stress, etc., producing characteristic symptoms; illness or sickness in general" (Dictionary.com, 2007).

The main point of several of these definitions is that they are defining disease. As pointed out in *Depathologizing Psychopathology* (Wasserman & Wasserman, 2016), we are overreaching and incorrectly including responses to stress as medically defined mental illness or disease. As McNally (2011) points out, there is increasing difficulty in distinguishing "mental disorders" from "mental distress." He goes on to highlight that these everyday problems that cause stress are being turned into medical disorders requiring medical intervention. NCLT rejects this blanket idea of a "disease causing agent" causing a need for medical intervention, and for that reason NCLT therapists often avoid using the term when they are discussing problems associated with learning which has become maladaptive. Remember that learning is based on synaptic changes which are affected by the products of specific genes expressed under specific conditions. Learning, therefore, is the product of a consistent and ongoing interaction between the individual's experiences and their genetically derived predispositions, a process termed epigenetics (Elman et al., 1996). For NCLT, it is learning that has become maladaptive that is the process of psychotherapy.

In contrast to the "disease" model, the word disorder reduces the reliance on explanation through a physiological etiology. In medical usage it means "an abnormal physical or mental condition" (Merriam Webster, 2016) or a derangement or abnormality of function; a morbid physical or mental state (The Free Dictionary, 2016). The term is more acceptable to some because it stresses deviance from the accepted normal. It is commonly perceived to be relativistic in nature.

Lastly, as an appropriate segue into our next section, NCLT prefers to talk about mental health rather than mental illness.

Adaptation

NCLT stresses adaptation and that is why you will see the words adaptive and maladaptive used frequently in this book. Adaptation is defined as a change, or the process of change by which an organism or species becomes better suited to its environment. When you have problems of adaptation, you have problems in being successful in meeting the challenges of everyday life. From a mental health perspective, this implies that the outcome of the learning that produced a complicated, integrated, combined emotional and behavioral response does not produce successful adaptation to the environment in which the individual currently finds themselves. More specifically, the individual is not successful in resolving problems and challenges found in that environment. If, when you encounter problems, you successfully adapt, that means you have made changes or solutions that are "suitable to requirements or conditions; (You) adjust or modify fittingly" (Dictionary.com, 2007). These terms closely align with the process of relearning that characterizes NCLT treatment. In sum, NCLT is about taking behaviors (emotions etc.) which were adaptive at one point, but became overlearned and maladaptive, and teaching the client how to learn new strategies which are currently adaptive.

NCLT Practice Teaches the Model

The practice of NCLT also differs from most other therapeutic practice models in that NCLT therapists actively teach the model as part of the treatment. We do this because we want the client to "take over" the process of behavioral and emotional assessment and reformulation from us. One of the main reasons this is promoted is because NCLT is an educational process based on a model of mental health that stresses the developmental and learning nature of the outcome. Most mental health practice is based on a cure model; A doctor or practitioner cures the disease. That means they make it go away. The patient's involvement in the process is limited to compliance with the medical regimen. You don't have to understand how an antiviral works you just need to know that if you follow the regimen the virus will not be there. NCLT is different. The client understands why a particular technique is being utilized, how that technique will work, and what the expected outcome will be. Not only does the NCLT therapist understand how a disorder of mental health would develop, they articulate that knowledge to their clients. This is done so that the clients develop automaticity as to the identification of problems and the development of adaptive responses. In this way, the clients can both learn to avoid the same pitfalls in the future and assist in the identification and de-automization of existing triggers to maladaptive behavior everyday instead of waiting to come to the therapist's office. This both expedites the initial process of change and serves as an "inoculation" of knowledge designed to forestall problems in the future.

Ultimately, therefore, you know you are an NCLT therapist if you accept the theory of the development of mental health that NCLT is founded upon. That foundation principle alone sets NCLT apart from many of the models of therapeutic intervention that are currently in use. Accepting that model as a foundation for your therapy sets you, as an NCLT therapist, apart from other therapists.

NCLT Practice Is Eclectic in Tool Selection and Specific in Model

Many types of therapeutic interventions are appropriate for use within an NCLT model as long as their utilization is designed to achieve a specific outcome related to the overall model of the development of mental health that NCLT is based upon. NCLT is not eclecticism. Rather, what this means is that therapeutic procedures are selected based upon their ability to affect the target and that this selection is informed by empirically based research that supports the selection. For example, a number of techniques could be selected to address anxiety related to a specific life event of a patient. They would all be valid for use as long as they met the following criteria:

1. The specific trigger for the targeted response is identified. It is entirely likely that one trigger will serve as the starting point for a similar response in a variety of circumstances for which the response has been generalized.
2. A target goal has been selected and an operationally defined outcome measure identified.
3. The reason for the expected outcome is explained to the client. This is a critically important step in NCLT practice because it is a learning-based environment. The client must understand how what is being done is expected to help so that they can use the same procedures themselves in order to generalize the behavior. For example, it does not make sense for the therapist to help the client relax in the face of an anxiety producing stimulus if at the same time the client does not learn to use the technique by themselves in future circumstances.
4. The intervention utilized has specific procedures built in that would allow for generalization and practice.

The Practice of Therapy

As we have pointed out elsewhere about many of the constructs that are central to the clinical practice of psychology, the definition of the construct of therapeutic practice has been very elusive (Friedman, 1988). Friedman does point out that any practice of psychotherapy must be able to address two central questions:

1. How does the therapist select what they will attend to?
2. What meaning does the client give to the therapist's selection?

NCLT has very specific answers to each of these questions.

How Does an NCLT Therapist Select to What They Will Attend?

An NCLT therapist is always looking for clusters of responses and the triggers for those clusters. For example, keeping in mind that an NCLT therapist would view anxiety as a highly developed schema, derived from a hyper aroused flight response and generalized to many situations by learned interaction, the NCLT therapist would spend time learning about the environmental triggers that were productive of the maladaptive anxiety based response. The therapist would not need to identify all of the triggers. In reality just a few triggers would be sufficient to get started with the training. As we have detailed elsewhere in this volume, the adaptive responses would be paired with the environmentally based trigger and opportunities for practice identified and described. In later sessions it is highly likely that the clients will detail other anxious responses and new triggers for which the newly learned response set could be generalized.

What Meaning Does the Client Give to the Therapists' Selection?

The NCLT therapy model, differently from some other interventions, is active in ascribing meaning or significance to the selected therapeutic target. That is because it is a directed, learning-based model that requires the client to understand why things are being done and what outcome is expected. As we have indicated, the meaning we wish the patient to derive is the identification of the triggers and the role these triggers play in evoking the learned automated maladaptive responses they wished to change when they entered therapy. This requires that the client has awareness of the NCLT model of mental health development. This awareness is provided to the client as an outline in the first session in order to form the elementary scaffold upon which future learning is based.

What Are the Characteristics of a Good Therapist in General and Which of Them Describes the Strength of NCLT in Specific?

NCLT is a model of the development of adaptive emotional and behavioral adaptation. Treatment practice occurs within the parameters acknowledged by most psychotherapies. There are well-researched behaviors that characterize the conduct of successful psychotherapists (Whitbourne, 2011). These can be summarized as follows:

1. **Possession of a sophisticated set of interpersonal skills.**
   Psychotherapists who are able to express themselves well and are clearly understandable to their clients are effective. Other skills that improve effectiveness are the ability to sense what other people are thinking and feeling, and to demonstrate empathy with their client's perspectives.
2. **Ability to help you feel you can trust the therapist.**
   Effective therapists are those whose clients believe that their therapists will be helpful because the therapist communicates both verbally and nonverbally that they are someone the client can trust.
3. **Willingness to establish an alliance with you.**
   One of the strongest predictors of a good therapeutic outcome is the client's perception that they are in a partnership with their therapists. Effective therapists are able to form these therapeutic alliances with many types of patients. NCLT therapists stress the teaching aspects of these alliances. There is a learning partnership established to explore the patterns of adaptation and maladaptation, and then work done cooperatively to improve adaptation.
4. **Ability to provide an explanation of your symptoms and can adapt this explanation as circumstances change.**

Clients want to know why they're experiencing their symptoms and what you are going to do to help them. As we have seen this is a particular strength of NCLT due to its emphasis on having clients understand and learn the mechanics of behavior and emotional change.

5. **Commitment to developing a consistent and acceptable treatment plan.**

   Effective therapists conduct an assessment very early in treatment. Following that assessment, they should develop a treatment plan and share that treatment plan with you. As we have seen in NCLT assessment begins almost as soon as the client enters the room for the first time. In addition it is continuous over the course of treatment with modifications occurring regularly as the learning and related behavioral and emotional regulation changes occur.

6. **Communication of confidence about the course of therapy.**

   As NCLT is an evidence-based model with a strong research validated (for its component parts) foundation, NCLT therapists are able to communicate to clients the belief that therapy will be worthwhile. This allows their clients to feel secure in the knowledge that the therapists know what they're doing, and why.

7. **Attention to the progress of therapy and communication of this interest to the client.**

   NCLT therapists, as most good therapists, are interested in finding out how their clients are responding to treatment. They show that they expect their clients to improve and why.

8. **Flexibility in adapting treatment to the particular client's characteristics.**

   A good therapist recognizes their strengths and limitations. In addition, they recognize that some treatments are better than others for particular psychological issues. They recognize that they must make accommodations for the client's particular characteristics. NCLT is particularly suited in this regard because, as an integrated model, it permits the inclusion of many types of techniques

9. **Inspiration of hope and optimism about your chances of improvement.**

   Although this was the original description of this trait we prefer the statement belief and a strong conviction about the possibility of improvement. In NCLT this stems from the model that indicates that many of these maladaptive behaviors are learned and as a result that they can be unlearned.

10. **Sensitivity toward your client's culture, personal values, and background.**

    Effective therapists demonstrate respect for the culture, values, and backgrounds of their clients. NCLT therapists are no different from any other therapist in this regard.

11. **Possession of self-insight.**

    An effective therapist is self-aware and is able to separate his or her own issues from those of clients.

12. **Reliance on the best research evidence.**

    Effective therapists stay current with the latest developments in clinical psychology, particularly in their areas of expertise. They alter the selection of treatment methodology to be consistent with the latest knowledge. This, perhaps, is one of the greatest strengths of NCLT. It is dependent on current research and is flexible enough to change if new research indicates a different procedure may be more efficacious than existing models. As an integrative model, new therapy techniques can be instantly and seamlessly adaptive. This is because NCLT is not technique specific but theory specific.

13. **Involvement in continued training and education.**
NCLT therapists are committed to continuous quality improvement and development of the model.

As we indicated all of these characteristics are not the exclusive purview of NCLT therapists, but can be found in all effective therapists whatever their chosen model. Given NCLT research and learning foundations they are intimately enmeshed in everyday NCLT practice.

Insight Is Not Enough

An NCLT therapist recognizes that insight alone is not sufficient for therapeutic progress to occur. Lange and Jakubowski (1973) made this case succinctly in their book "Responsible Assertive Behavior." They noted that when a person becomes more assertive through simple insight or encouragement on the part of the therapist, that person has only been exposed to the concept of assertion. In order to acquire the training required to actually engage in assertive behavior, practice of the desired behavior was necessary.

An NCLT therapist understands that consistent practice of both the new cognitive construct and the related behavior is essential for the acquisition of a new skill set that represents new clusters of responses in reaction to new triggers.

Lange and Jakubowski also point out that the application of a therapeutic technique is enhanced when it is tailored to meet the individual client's circumstances. In NCLT terms this implies that the therapist recognizes that the patterns of related stimuli that comprise an individual's reaction are idiosyncratic to that person based upon their history.

NCLT also recognizes that the improvement of the effectiveness of psychotherapy may best be accomplished by learning to improve one's ability to relate to clients and tailoring that relationship to individual clients (Lambert & Barley, 2001). They note that "decades of research indicate that the provision of therapy is an interpersonal process in which a main curative component is the nature of the therapeutic relationship. Clinicians must remember that this is the foundation of our efforts to help others" (p. 357).

We would want to point out that just because this has been historically correct, it does not imply that it has to be an accurate characterization of future therapeutic endeavors. The inherent problems with the sensitivity and specificity of therapeutic practice may have resulted in the current reality of nonspecific treatment effects being the most important variable, but as therapies become more targeted and more responsive to how the brain processes the information learned in therapy, specific treatment effects from the treatments themselves can reasonably be expected. In fact, this outcome is to be desired. In medicine it would hardly be optimal if the primary determiner of outcome was how well you got along with your doctor, not the medicine you were prescribed or the surgery you undertook.

Psychotherapy Integration and NCLT

There is recognition that most forms of psychotherapy share a group of common factors. This term refers to those aspects of psychotherapy that are found in most models of therapy. These aspects and techniques cut across all theoretical lines and are present in most psychotherapeutic activities. These common factors integrate psychotherapeutic practice on a functional level. While there is no standard list of common factors, the following will serve as an exemplar:

- a therapeutic alliance established between the patient and the therapist
- exposure of the patient to prior difficulties, either in imagination or in reality
- a new corrective emotional experience that allows the patient to experience past problems in new and more benign ways
- expectations by both the therapist and the patient that positive change will result from the treatment
- therapist qualities, such as attention, empathy, and positive regard, that are facilitative of change in treatment
- the provision by the therapist to the patient of a reason for the problems that are being experienced

As we have seen NCLT practice includes all of these aspects. There are a number of ways that the practice of therapy can be integrated (Psychotherapy Integration, 2016).

The first is the common factors method described above. There are three other ways:

Assimilative Integration
In this approach, the therapist has a preference to one particular theoretical approach, but is willing to incorporate techniques from other therapeutic approaches. This approach reflects the general belief in psychotherapy practice that there is no one approach to therapy that is appropriate for every patient.

Technical Eclecticism
Technical Eclecticism is really a form of Assimilative Integration where there is no unifying theoretical models that underlie the approach. It is the most common form of eclecticism among those practitioners who term themselves as eclectic. The therapist relies on previous experience, clinical expertise, and knowledge of the theoretical and research literature to choose interventions that are appropriate for the patient.

The NCLT Way: Theoretical Integration

The fourth and most difficult way to integrate therapy practice is called "Theoretical Integration." This approach demands the integration of theoretical concepts from different approaches that may differ in their fundamental philosophy about human behavior. Theoretical Integration tries to bring together those theoretical approaches themselves, and then to develop a comprehensive unifying theory integrating them all. To date, psychology has not produced a unifying theory of practice that meets these criterion but, NCLT at least appears to do so in that it provides a model of development of mental health that will allow for the use of all major systems therapy when used within the context of the model.

NCLT Therapists Understand that the Therapeutic Relationship Is Valuable

Nothing about what we have already said should be construed to mean that an NCLT therapist would claim that the model and technique are so powerful that they did not have to worry about the relationship that they worked on between themselves and their clients. That would be as inaccurate for psychotherapy as it would be inaccurate for medicine. There is ample research to suggest that the quality of the therapeutic relationship remains a crucial variable contributing to beneficial outcome. For example, a therapist's qualities such flexibility, honesty, respectfulness, trustworthiness, confidence, warmth, interest, and openness were found to contribute positively to the creation, maintenance, and effectiveness of the therapeutic relationship. In addition, techniques such as exploration, reflection, noting past therapy success, accurate interpretation, facilitating the expression of affect, and attending to the patient's experience also contributed to the effectiveness of the relationship (Ackerman & Hilsenroth, 2003).

How Do You Know When Your Work Is Done?

The traditional idea of cure must refer to the concept of disease/disorder in order to understand it. Psychology has always had a somewhat bifurcated relationship with the idea of cure as an outcome. Take this statement from the American Psychological Association regarding the treatment for anxiety: "The large majority of people who suffer from an anxiety disorder are able to reduce or eliminate their anxiety symptoms and return to normal functioning after several months of appropriate psychotherapy" (American Psychological Association, 2016). This seems to imply that treatment is done when the symptoms of anxiety are no longer an issue for the client. Contrast that statement with this one from the exact same source "No one plan works well for all patients. Treatment needs to be tailored to the needs of the patient and to the type of disorder, or disorders, from which the individual suffers."

This latter statement seems to imply that there is something larger than the symptoms that at play; The disorder itself, that causes the anxiety, is cured.

It might surprise you to learn that there is not a great deal of clarity as regards the end of treatment in the psychological literature. One website we reviewed had a section entitled "Tips for starting therapy" but did not have a corresponding section entitled tips for ending therapy. "One of the challenges faced by people who have a mental illness — such as depression, bipolar disorder, schizophrenia, or ADHD or the like — is that not too many people will talk to you about 'curing' the condition. (Except snake-oil salesmen, who will claim they can cure your bipolar disorder with their amazing technique or CD.) In fact, you'd be hard-pressed to find a professional who talks openly about "cures" for mental illness" (Grohol, 2009). Mental health people are so averse to talking about cure that we have borrowed a code word from the lexicon of non-curable, but manageable diseases. We use the term in remission. Standard practice in the field is to append the term in remission to the diagnosis when we close a case or treatment ends.

NCLT takes a symptom-based approach to the termination of treatment. In brief, when the symptoms that caused you to seek treatment are no longer present, treatment is concluded. This sentiment was echoed by Friedman (2007) who stated "the term 'cure,' I think, is illusory - even undesirable- because there will always be problems to repair. Having no problems is an unrealistic goal. It's more important for patients to be able to deal with their problems, and to handle adversity, when it inevitably arises" (p. F6).

There is more, however, and the following represents a good compilation of accomplishments that an NCLT practitioner would consider representative of a completed course of treatment (adapted from (WebMD, 2016):

- the client is able to understand the behaviors, emotions, and ideas that contribute to behavior and learn how to modify them
- the client is able to understand and identify the life problems or events that contribute to the difficulty and understand which of those problems he/she may be able to solve or improve and which they can safely ignore
- The client regains a sense of control and pleasure in life
- The client eliminates maladaptive responses to target stimuli and learn adaptive coping techniques and problem-solving skills
- The client can, in a developmentally appropriate manner, articulate the model that determined how these changes were accomplished

References

Ackerman, S., & Hilsenroth, M. (2003). A review of therapist characteristics and techniques positively impacting the therapeutic alliance. *Clinical Psychology Review, 23*(1), 1–33.

American Psychological Association. (2016). *Anxiety disorders and effective treatment*. Retrieved from American Psychological Association: http://www.apa.org/helpcenter/anxiety-treatment.aspx

Dictionary.com. (2007). *Disease*. Retrieved from Dictionary.com: http://www.dictionary.com/browse/disease

Elman, J., Bates, E., Johnson, M., Karmiloff-Smith, A., Parisi, D., & Plunkett, K. (1996). *Rethinking innateness: a connectionist perspective on development*. Cambridge, MA: MIT Press.

The Free Dictionary. (2016). *Disorder*. Retrieved from The Free Dictionary: http://medical-dictionary.thefreedictionary.com/disorder

Friedman, L. (1988). *The anatomy of psychotherapy*. Hillsdale, NJ: Analytic Press.

Friedman, T. (2007, October 30). How to figure out when therapy is over. *The New York Times*, p. F6.

Grohol, J. (2009, May 26). *How do you cure mental illness?* Retrieved from World of Psychology: http://psychcentral.com/blog/archives/2009/05/22/how-do-you-cure-mental-illness/

Lambert, M., & Barley, D. (2001). Research summary on the therapeutic relationship and psychotherapy outcome. *Psychotherapy: Theory, Research, Practice, Training, 38*(4), 357–361. doi:10.1037/0033-3204.38.4.357.

Lange, A., & Jakubowski, P. (1973). *Responsive assertive behavior*. Champaign, IL: Research Press.

McNally, R. (2011). *What is mental illness?* Boston, MA: Belknap Press.

Merriam Webster. (2016). *Disease*. Retrieved from Merriam Webster Dictionary: http://www.merriam-webster.com/dictionary/disease

Psychotherapy integration. (2016). Retrieved from Encyclopedia of Mental DIsorders: http://www.minddisorders.com/Ob-Ps/Psychotherapy-integration.html

Robbins, M. (1992). Psychoanalytic and biological approaches to mental illness: Schizophrenia. *Journal of the American Psychoanalytic Association, 40*(2), 425–454.

Wasserman, T., & Wasserman, L. (2016). *Depathologizing psychopathology*. New York: Springer.

WebMD. (2016). *Mental health and psychotherapy*. Retrieved from WebMD: http://www.webmd.com/anxiety-panic/guide/mental-health-psychotherapy

Whitbourne, S. (2011, August 8). *13 qualities to look for in an effective psychotherapist*. Retrieved from Psychology Today: https://www.psychologytoday.com/blog/fulfillment-any-age/201108/13-qualities-look-in-effective-psychotherapist

Chapter 9
NCLT Therapy: Introductory Considerations

When a client comes for NCLT treatment, a good deal of the structure of the process of treatment intervention falls on the therapist. Therefore, is it a good idea to have a template of how the therapy process plays out over the series of sessions you have available. The average number of psychotherapy sessions for major depressive disorder in a community mental health environment averages about eight (Connolly-Gibbons et al., 2011). That means that you won't have a lot of time to accomplish your task, and that you must therefore plan to be very efficient. For us, this also implies that the more we can teach a client how to manage their own problems going forward, the greater the long range impact our intervention will have. This is very much akin to the saying "Give a man a fish, he will eat for a day. Teach him *how* to fish…".

Before the First Session

Even before an NCLT therapist meets the person coming in for treatment, the therapist performs some preparatory steps. Remember, NCLT is an integrative therapeutic approach which incorporates a person's neurophysiological integrity with their behavior, feelings and thoughts, and inherently, with the symptoms bringing them to therapy. This has important implications for the role of theory for an NCLT therapist. Most psychotherapists have a complex and changeable relationship with the theories that underlie their work. Research has suggested that theory was generally important to psychotherapists in an abstract sense. However, research regarding the therapist's use of theory indicates that psychotherapists may construct and renegotiate their relationships to theory through conversations with others (Osborne, 2015). This suggests that the role of theory in a pragmatic sense, as utilized in clinical practice, is somewhat less than a scientific template and somewhat more like a

© Springer International Publishing AG 2017   101
T. Wasserman, L.D. Wasserman, *Neurocognitive Learning Therapy: Theory and Practice*, DOI 10.1007/978-3-319-60849-5_9

negotiated settlement with contributions from interested parties. NCLT is quite different. The NCLT therapist prepares for the first session by re-familiarizing themselves with the models' basic tenets and rules which are solidly grounded in research of learning theory, probabilistic reward calculations, and memory reconsolidation. In addition, they will make sure that they understand the relationship of any type of preferred intervention they may have to the core principles of the model. Of course we do not expect any therapist to sit down and review tomes of material. We do expect that the therapist will be able to frame their questions and hypotheses in a manner consistent with NCLT theory. That would include being able to ask "How" questions rather than often unanswerable why questions or closed ended yes/no questions. For example, we would want to know how well the client tolerates stress, frustration, etc. How is this person feeling, thinking, handling emotional regulation, etc. How is this person perpetuating the issue.

As a temporal step, we would peruse the rather extensive intake form we have clients complete before arriving at our office. This information is gathered to obtain an initial assessment of the possible contributions of history, current relationships, schooling ,and medical problems. Please keep in mind that NCLT has both connectionist and constructivist roots, and we are going to be spending time looking at the various contributions of all aspects of the environment and the constitutional neuropsychology that determined the functionality of the connectome. For example, how is this person's recent history, home life, medications, etc., contributing to their presentation.

When the Client First Arrives

When the new client arrives, the first thing that an NCLT therapist has to ascertain is the reason the client is there. This does not mean a general description or asking the rather self-answering question "Why did you come for therapy" but rather implies an attempt to obtain some specificity about the referral issues that brought the client to the office. This is a somewhat different process from many other models in that the therapist is going to help the client understand the schema by which they are operating. This may include the client's means of processing information obtained from stimuli in their environment. This discussion introduces the idea that external information is processed through internally mediated schemas (often at this point referred to as filters). A stated goal of therapy will include teaching the clients to have a healthy respect for their own biological predispositions and how their response patterns are contributing to both their healthy and maladaptive patterns of responses. In this way intervention begins almost immediately in that follow-up questions to the identification of various situations and the individual's responses frequently seek to determine the emotional/behavioral triggers from the beginning. For example, if a person indicates that they are depressed, a second question might be "How do you know?," or "How are you experiencing that?" This is a question asking about what physiological, cognitive, and emotional triggers the person is associating with the identified mood state, and likely significant clues as to how and where to target your interventions.

The Role of History Taking in NCLT Practice

As is true of so many things in the world of psychotherapy, there is little consensus and scant empirical evidence to support a position on the role of history taking in psychotherapy. Some schools advocate extensive history taking designed to help the therapist understand the various historical and environmental influences that have shaped the person. Other schools "dive right in" focusing on solutions to current problems that the client is facing. History taking, in some sense, is as much a reflection of the need of the therapist as it is a requirement for a good beginning to a therapy process. That being said, NCLT has a position on history taking. The goal of history taking is specific to the trigger or schema under discussion. The goal is twofold. In part, the goal is to identify all of the elements that the client associates with the particular schema in question. This is done in an attempt to identify as many of the triggers as you can that produce the undesirable response pattern. You will never get them all. At first you will get the most obvious or most strongly associated ones and that is all you need to get started. The second goal of history taking is to help determine an alternative conceptualization of the presenting problem. One that is consistent with the presenting issues from a life course model perspective. As the sessions branch out from the first, more topics will be covered, more schemas identified, and a more comprehensive history of the person relative to their maladaptive response patterns will emerge. The procedure is similar to mind mapping. Here is a map of the client Melissa whom we will speak about in detail later. It was begun during the first session and completed over several additional sessions.

Additional Considerations in the First Sessions

The Need to Diagnose

Mental health professionals have been subject to the insurance labeling and diagnosis protocols for so long, that we expect that the client is going to present with something that is diagnosable. We are required to have that assumption because the rules of the road mandate that the person has to have a diagnosable condition in order for insurance to cover their treatment. In many cases we have to provide the diagnosis before we do anything else. A resulting second assumption is that our job is to find out what this diagnosis is, and then perform some treatment to ameliorate

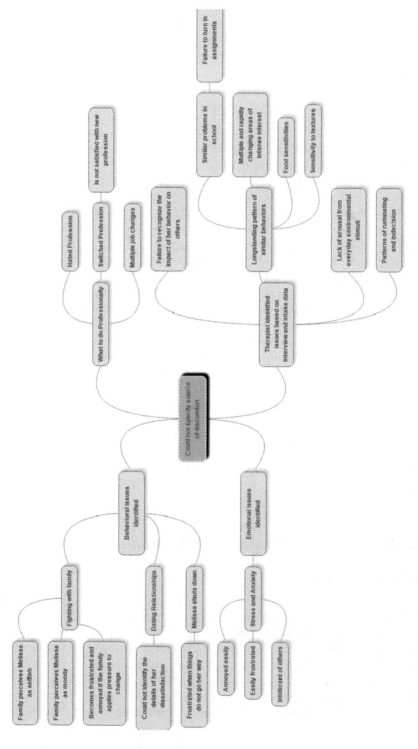

Created with MindMup at www.mindmup.com

the symptomology related to the particular diagnosis we have assigned. This is a problem endemic in metal health practice today. According to Psych Central "nobody likes to admit this, but without a diagnosis, the therapist won't get paid by your insurance company. And it can't just be any diagnosis (despite the mental health parity law passed last year). It has to be a "covered" disorder. This means that if a client comes in to therapy with something that isn't quite clinical depression, a therapist may diagnose it anyway, so that the session will be reimbursed. (That's one of the many reasons why you shouldn't put too much faith into your diagnosis in the first place)" (Grohol, 2009).

We covered many of the issues related to diagnoses in our first book (Wasserman & Wasserman, 2016) and will not review them here. Suffice it to say that we do not endorse this practice and that neither of these assumptions are an absolute mandate for NCLT. While there might be a diagnosable condition that is understandable according to the NCLT model of mental health, the model that NCLT proposes considers it possible that the client is not happy with the way that they are thinking, feeling, or behaving and wish to change some aspect of it. They may simply recognize that some aspect of their behavior is maladaptive and wish to change it. In fact, that may be a diagnosis of mental health! It is our job to help them understand how their individual constellation of neurophysiology and psychological responsivity interplay, creating schemas, and to help them make corrections to their system so that they are more resilient and adaptive.

Creating the Diagnosis Does Not End the Process of Determining What Your Client Needs

What we mean by this is that we recognize that a diagnosis may be necessary for insurance, or simply for legal and ethical compliance. That is a reality of our field. However, what we mean to make clear is that, for example, a diagnosis of anxiety does not conclude the NCLT process. It is not enough to simply state that a client is anxious. It is also not sufficient to say that you are treating anxiety. It is important to understand the anxiety as a precipitant to the behavior with which it occurs. These occur in tandem, and should be treated that way. We recognize that anxiety can be treated psychopharmacologically. While it may be sometimes true that reducing the anxiety by means of medication will impact the automated and learned association between the anxiety response and the trigger, it is also sometimes true that medication is taken after the anxiety response has been triggered and merely serves to dampen the intensity of the anxiety. In either event, the attribution that the client learns is that the medication is what "cured" the anxiety. This is not always desirable. It is true that under some conditions anti-anxiety medication may have diminished the level of anxiety temporarily and allowed for the connection between the anxiety and a particular trigger to be weakened. This is in effect desensitization and it is a well-known and effective behavior modification process. One could see, for example, the benefit of an anti-anxiety medication for the occasional flyer. It is also possible, and is frequently seen in therapy, wherein a client states that they were becoming very anxious and "needed" their anti-anxiety pill. Doesn't this in fact reinforce the concept of their lack of control, thereby further reinforcing the notion that they are not competent, resilient, etc.? It would be preferable, according to the NCLT model, that the client understand what was transpiring so that they understood that the connection can be modulated in this and other ways, and that they themselves can control that process if they choose to. We believe that it is preferable for the client to attribute the more adaptive physiological response pattern to their own control and behavioral efforts as opposed to becoming psychologically dependent on an outside agent.

That is why NCLT is theory driven. NCLT intervention requires the therapist to have an understanding of the person's own neurophysiological predispositions, the etiology and the specification of the triggers, and specific behavioral and emotional response patterns within a life course model; the schemas they have created.

With respect to the application of interventions, NCLT stresses that mental illness is not a prerequisite for maladaptive behavior to occur. Nor should one assume that any particular patient will be best served by the application of any therapist's preferred treatment approach. This is not to say that we should not have a preferred model of treatment, but it is to say that no one preferred model of traditional treatment will usually be sufficient to handle most issues that confront us across the idiosyncrasies of any particular patient. In fact, rigid adherence to one treatment orientation may result in missing the foundations which are maintaining the schema.

Sometimes Just the Knowledge Helps

NCLT holds that information is power. There is the possibility, and not infrequently the case, that the sharing of the foundational information we offer may help a client understand how they are thinking, and may in and of itself be sufficient for the client to initiate change. We have increasingly found that once we explain things like memory reconsolidation, gating, and reward valence to clients, that they are able to apply these constructs to many of the problems that they are dealing with, and that the application of the more pedantic elements of the traditional therapeutic approaches are not required.

As opposed to some approaches that assess the clients' functional capacity and goodness of fit within a preferred model of treatment, an NCLT therapist has to assess each client individually based upon their reason for seeking therapy, their symptomology and how those symptoms were acquired and maintained. The job of an NCLT therapist is to assess the schema that forms the basis of their client's symptomology.

Some Initial Considerations About Our Initial Considerations

One of the other main points NCLT has been stressing is our problem with diagnoses and the behavioral descriptors of diagnoses. We appreciate the diagnostic "shorthand," but forcing us to diagnose a person sometimes is misleading. Take a moment and think about your role as clinician and diagnoses. If someone comes to you utilizing their insurance, you will, of course, need to provide an insurance code and that insurance code is an affirmation of your belief that a client has an illness that requires treatment.

Typically, that is what we all at first do. We attempt to determine which disorder our new client has. How do you determine which diagnosis you would to choose? What if, as we shall soon see in the case of Melissa, the individual is not particularly depressed or anxious? What if they do not fit the requirements of a personality disorder? You go on to ask how impaired is Melissa? Does Melissa present with symptomology sufficient to assert that she is pathological? Is she rigid enough to call her a Type A personality? Obsessive compulsive? ADHD? Is she impulsive? Think about how your choice of a diagnosis will affect your treatment direction. Remember, that your work may be scrutinized to determine how your treatment impacted the "mental illness" you just gave her.

An Important Side Note

In case you are just glossing over the importance of the preceding statement, take a moment and consider this, because this happens more frequently than you may think: Mrs. Sally Smith comes to see you while using her husband's employer sponsored insurance to help pay for the sessions. She is distressed about her marriage and her perceived derogatory comments about her parenting from her husband. After a while the couple decides to divorce. A rather bitter custody dispute ensues. As part of the divorce strategy the husband, Mr. Smith, citing your diagnosis, uses it as the basis for a claim that Melissa is too emotionally unstable to parent their two young children. He thereby petitions for full parental custody and for supervised visitation for Mrs. Smith when she has visitation with the couple's young children. How would you explain your diagnosis in a court of law?

In order to circumvent this possibility and avoid the use of a potential damaging label, the most logical thing to do is to decide to avoid the issue altogether by trying to say that Mrs. Smith is fine. It is just that she is having a transitory problem adjusting to stress. You would not be alone. One of the most frequently used diagnoses to handle just such situations is Adjustment Disorder. Depending on the study involved, between 25 and 50% of all psychiatric patients are identified with this particular disorder. But is it really a disorder? The field still lacks data about its rightful place as a clinical entity. As Carta, Balestrieri, Murru, and Hardoy (2009) indicate, this may be caused by a difficulty in facing, with purely descriptive methods, a "pathogenic label," based on a stressful event, for which a subjective impact has to be considered. Adjustment disorder has been classified as being as vague and all-encompassing as to be useless as a functional description of a disease. It continues, however, to serve a useful clinical purpose for clinicians seeking a non-stigmatizing label for patients who need a diagnosis for insurance coverage of therapy. In other words, we use it to label something that is not a disorder, *as* a disorder/illness, albeit one with less repercussions, so that the patient can get the necessary support to pay for our services, which they need for mental health reasons. This not only renders the predictability of the diagnosis limited as far as treatment is concerned, it clearly demonstrates the limitations of the medical model when it comes to addressing the mental health needs of many of our clients.

Case Example

When trying to understand a process, it is often useful to have a case exemplar to study how the system works in real time. It is for this reason that we are going to present several cases which represent composites of typically seen clients and scenarios in clinical practice. We hope to utilize these scenarios to encompass a wide range of issues that demonstrate the similarities and differences between NCLT and other therapeutic approaches. We are going to do this by presenting the case information, having a discussion of the various aspects of the model that led to the treatment formulation and then outlining the treatment formulation. At relevant points we may include research that supports the NCLT model's conceptualization.

Melissa

Melissa is a 29-year-old, single, college graduate with an architect degree. Melissa presented with a Reason for Referral of "----------------------". This is not a misprint. Many of the people who come for initial consultations do not provide their reasons on the form, or cannot encapsulate them in a short statement. While on the intake form the reason for referral was left blank, one section of the intake form asks clients to rank the concerns that brought them to treatment from a list of possible issues, such as financial, relationships, family, or sexual issues. While Melissa was not able to verbally clarify her reason for coming, she was able to check off several areas of difficulty so that an initial starting point could be determined. Melissa identified stress, anxiety, family and relationship issues as areas of primary concern.

Therapeutic Consideration 1 In actuality, some initial impression was possible from these few snippets of information. Melissa was not able to express or summarize what brought her to the office, although she was able to indicate the presence of issues when they were provided on a form for her to check off. This is an interesting point in that she would not or could not articulate or express what brought her to treatment, although she clearly knew the areas of concern she had. Another possibility is that she did not want to take the time to write them down. This issue will also reemerge later. As we will see later, these behaviors were not uncommon for Melissa. In addition, the form asks that the client rate, on a scale of one to ten, the seriousness of any of the issues identified. Interestingly, Melissa rated each of the areas she identified as a "5." Whether this indicated initial defensiveness, the fact that Melissa may have only one moderate level of emotional response, or that she had come to therapy because she was only mildly upset about a few things remained to be clarified.

Returning to Melissa Melissa entered the office as an attractive, well dressed 29 year old. She reported the following: She is well educated, having achieved her degree in architecture. She worked for 2 years at an architectural firm in a major metropolitan city, which specialized in commercial buildings. Melissa discovered that she did not like the architectural world, nor the city in the north east where she was living. She left the firm, and the city in which she worked, and moved back to her home state where she opened her own jewelry store.

When questioned about her choice of career in architecture, Melissa indicated that she chose it because she likes designing things. Melissa also reported that her mother, whose opinion Melissa respected, didn't think architecture would be a good choice. But Melissa liked the challenges posed by new designs, and so she went ahead with her academic and professional plan. She enjoyed working in architecture for a while, but lost interest as the projects lacked creativity, representing what she called "cookie cutter" designs. Opening a jewelry shop allowed Melissa to be creative and showcase her own designs. While this allowed Melissa to express her creativity, Melissa indicated that the rent for the jewelry store was high and that she was not earning enough to cover her costs.

As the clinician, you establish that Melissa has no history of drug or alcohol abuse. Her childhood was accomplished without incident. She attended several private schools. Her medical history is negative in that she had no prior history of treatment for a major disease, was not on any medication and did not have a prior history of working with a therapist secondary to mental health concerns.

Interpersonally, Melissa maintains close, but somewhat tumultuous, relationships with her parents, sister, and brother. After some discussion of this report it becomes clear that the family members are concerned about a pattern of behavior that they believe represents a problem, and that the tumultuous relationships Melissa describes with them are the result of the family repeatedly expressing their concerns regarding aspects of Melissa's behavior. Melissa reports that the family is concerned about the fact that she cannot find satisfaction in her work, waivers on where she wants to live, and has been in an "on again/off again" relationship with her current boyfriend Jeff. They tell her that they see her as moody and insensitive. Recently, for example, Melissa's mother went out of the way to prepare a special Thanksgiving dinner for the family. Melissa reported that although aware of her mother's efforts, she ate quickly and retired to the guest room. In explaining her behavior to the therapist, Melissa indicated that when she left the room she was not angry or distressed in any way. Rather, that she had tired of the conversation quickly and preferred to watch a television program. Melissa reported that she was surprised that her mother and family were upset with her, and that it did not occur to her that her behavior would have the impact on the other people that it did. Melissa indicated that this was not the first incident of this sort to occur. She often bores of relationships quickly and will absent herself from conversations when the topic no longer interests her.

Therapeutic Consideration 2 Placing yourself in the role of the therapist, where would you go from here? Keeping in mind NCLT's life course orientation that dictates that physical, environmental, temperamental, and emotional factors are all determinants of behaviors, you might, as a good NCLT clinician, begin to ask Melissa details about her personal history. You are going to use this information to decide how to focus these sessions. But which details do you focus on, and why? From what, amongst all of this, do you choose to talk about?

If one is a relational therapist or has a psychodynamic or cognitive behavioral focus, the information gathered would be designed to answer treatment specific requirements. That is, one's preferred therapeutic model will determine how you filter the information. For example, as a cognitive behavior therapist you might frame the discussion to ascertain what demands Melissa was making on the other people in her environment, or what demands she perceived others to be making on her. As a relational therapist you might focus on her feelings regarding her poor relationships with her family members. As an analyst you might look for the root causes of these dysfunctional relationships. In many cases your preferred model would determine exactly what you would decide to talk about.

An NCLT therapist would do that as well, but places all of these influences on equal footing as regards contribution to the current pattern of adaptive (maladaptive) behavior. Instead of specific events, circumstances, or cognitions, an NCLT therapist is looking to identify the patterns and themes into which these events, circumstances, and cognitions fall. These patterns determine how an individual addresses the various problems that confront them. Remember, we have learned that humans pattern match, and the group with which the new event is pattern matched, determines the responses that event is likely to evoke. These themes and patterns are associated with the automated processes that determine Melisa's emotional and behavioral pattern of response. Given the life course orientation of the NCLT model, we recognize that the beginnings of these response patterns often occur early on in the individual's development, a fact which makes careful history taking around these central themes all the more important.

As an NCLT practitioner you are going to look at multiple areas of development including academic, developmental history, medical history and where in the life span this person is. You are going to keep in mind primacy; how does this person respond? Do they respond emotionally, viscerally, or cognitively? In actuality they respond in all these ways, but usually a person will have a preferred venue of response. So you are going to be looking at patterns of behavior and cognitive styles.

You Can't Get It All Done in the First Session

It should be pointed out that the gathering of a complete history is not necessarily accomplished in the first session, or even in the first several sessions. We do not want a client to spend the entire first session recounting their reasons for being distressed thus compounding, and in effect substantiating, the validity of their oft times maladaptive emotional response. We believe that a client should leave the first session with a reasonable and positive expectation of what is to transpire in therapy. In this sense, intervention begins immediately. Clients are told about some of the basic

NCLT concepts and the model is explained. As a result, we take enough history to form a reasonable hypothesis about what some of these central themes are and begin to work from there. Further discussions in collaboration with the client will determine the accuracy or inaccuracy of these initial conceptualization themes. It is a process of mutual exploration and definition between you and your client. Now back to Melissa…

Clarifying the Reason for Referral
As we have pointed out, one of the first requirements of the NCLT process is to clarify the various issues and the triggers that lead to their expression. So the therapist began the process of specifying both the reason for referral and the pertinent history that Melissa associated with these problems.

Returning to Melissa Melissa has dated several men, but she has had mainly two long-term relationships, including Jeff. She has always planned on getting married, and she is worried about her age and not being married. She cannot identify the reason why she hasn't found the "right one," but reports that she has never been really excited or "in love" with anyone. Her hobbies include hang gliding, rafting, travel, and gourmet food. Melissa returns to describing how her family is "always on her," asking hundreds of questions and "ganging up on her." She describes how when they do this, she just "shuts down." This in turn only makes them more annoyed.

Therapeutic Consideration 3 Melissa has now presented us with two potential clusters, or schemas, each rich in history and complex behavioral and emotional response patterns. The first set of clusters includes family, dating relationships, and professional concerns, all of which center around lack of engagement, underarousal, and lack of persistence. The second set of clusters involves Melissa's failure to recognize the impact of her behavior on others and her internal emotional responses. Taken together, these schemas suggest a pattern of impulsive decision making, lack of long-term planning and poor persistence.

Now take a moment and think about Melissa's pattern of behavior. Which diagnosis would you be considering at this point? Do you have enough information to consider any? Do you need more? What else would you need? These questions are pertinent if you believe your first job is to establish a diagnosis. If you believe that the only way to understand what troubles Melissa can be represented by a diagnostic conceptualization, this step is necessary. If that isn't necessary, then you can proceed to hypothesis testing and beginning the work.

Although the benefits of a selection-specific shorthand are obvious, a diagnosis based on constructs consisting of an amalgam of symptoms obliterates the unique nature of each client as regards the development of the connectome, the behavior that evolves from it, and their routine complex patterns of behavior which represent schema. In a very real way, diagnostic categories, as they currently exist, are the exact opposite of what NCLT is trying to accomplish. Rather than an amalgam of possibilities resulting in a global diagnosis, our job is to help Melissa understand the nature of her functioning. We are going to deconstruct the diagnostic descriptors and utilize only those which explain her functioning.

What forms a cohesive whole from the parts of the data is the idea that Melissa has difficulty regulating certain aspects of her executive function based upon issues related to arousal and reward valence. These particular areas of functioning include persistence as reflected in several job changes, and a history of starting projects and not finishing or sticking with them. As we have pointed out, these difficulties also involve impulse control, poor self-monitoring concerning the impact her behavior is having on others, poor planning, and poor organizing. All of this will become much clearer in the discussion of the second session.

Returning to Melissa During the discussion to this point the therapist took note of Melissa's communication style which consisted of incomplete expressions of thought, shifting from topic to topic and failing to completely explain an idea. When asked about this, Melissa reported that she had difficulty communicating the way that she felt about many things. She indicated that she became annoyed in conversation quickly, and that she often shut down. She reported that her parents complained that she rapidly became sullen and moody if she did not get her own way. They often labeled her selfish, a concept she found foreign in describing herself. Melissa, who despite this comment, perceived herself as being very close with her family, and was particularly upset about being labeled in this way.

In reviewing Melissa's verbal report to this point the therapist decided to get more information about the nature of the interactive problems between Melissa and her family. In response to additional questions, Melissa confirmed that the description matched what her family often complained about. She felt ganged up on during what she described as the family fights. She was often accused of being insensitive, and that the more she perceived herself as being attacked, the more quickly she shut down.

Therapeutic Consideration 4 Melissa had now added a history that indicated poor ability to organize her thoughts, poor ability to communicate her thoughts to others, and difficulty understanding the perspective of others, to the already provided descriptions of reduced emotional regulation and lack of arousal, engagement, and sustained effort with major self-selected life activities. These are all indicative of difficulty with the executive regulation of behavior, thought, and emotion that are often found in what many clinicians would consider representative of ADHH.

The NCLT model of ADHD (Wasserman & Wasserman, 2015) is quite different from the model represented in the DSM 5 (*Diagnostic and Statistical Manual of Mental Disorders*, 2013). NCLT posits that Attention Deficit Disorder represents an inefficiency of an integrated executive system, whose purpose is to allocate working memory to targeted tasks rather than the absence or dysfunction of a particular form of attention. A substantial portion of this inefficiency in the allocation of working memory represents poor engagement of the reward circuit with distinct circuits of learning and performance which control instrumental conditioning (learning). Efficient attention requires the interaction of these circuits. For most individuals who present with Attention Deficit Disorder, their problems represent the engagement, or lack thereof, of the motivational and reward circuit as opposed to problems, or disorders of attention traditionally defined as problems with orienting, focusing, and sustaining. In the NCLT model, attention is viewed as a gating function determined by novelty, flight or fight response, and reward history/valence affecting motivation.

As we noted above, we do not require that the entire history has to be taken in order to generate an initial hypothesis. Data collection from this point would either confirm or modify our initial impression, but the creation of a hypothesis provides a direction for further questioning. The initial hypothesis was that Melissa was presenting with executive function issues similar to those found in individuals with ADHD. Although Melissa presented with several areas to address in therapy, this hypothesis suggested that a unifying understanding of all of these issues would be found in understanding how effectively Melissa self-regulated and then integrated information.

It should also be noted that we have not said anything at this point that mentioned clinical disorder, pathology, or illness. Just because a person has difficulty with a particular function or task does not make that difficulty into an illness. On the whole, Melissa was successful and leading an adaptive life. She had completed a demanding academic program and received a degree in architecture. She was successfully employed in her career until she, herself, decided that she did not enjoy it enough to continue. Her relationships with men were successful and it was Melissa who decided that they weren't rewarding enough. Her unhappiness was her own, and her desire for understanding how these things were happening to her was the driving force behind her participation in therapy. The issue for NCLT is one of function, not illness.

Returning to Melissa After further discussion, Melissa reported that she went to a private High School because she excelled in golf and the school she went to permitted dual enrollment with a golf academy. She did not go on to play Golf in college. She completed her degree, a 5-year Bachelor of Architecture program, but did not like architecture and decided to change careers. Although she was academically successful she never really loved to read. She didn't rush home to do her assignments, but they got done. She reported that she enjoyed school athletics, particularly golf, and would play golf in preference to doing her homework. She never required academic accommodations. She reported that school was something one has to do, it was "a given" so to speak, and she did it.

Melissa also described that when she was in college she had to go to the library to find a quiet place to study. She indicated that she got easily distracted by noise and had difficulty sustaining attention as a result.

Completing the First Session: Introducing Elements of the Model
As we have indicated, NCLT likes to give the client a sample of the type of intervention that characterizes the process and provide a glimpse into the future course of treatment. For Melissa, this consisted of a brief introduction to the concept of the network organization of the brain and how executive function is defined in such a model. It was explained that these integrated networks were comprised of a number

of task specific activities, one of the main ones was the engagement of reward recognition systems that would produce arousal, engagement, and persistence. She was introduced to the concept of gating and the role of reward valuation in that process.

Melissa was specifically told that instead of interpreting her lack of interest and arousal as a characterological deficit, it might be more beneficial to think about these factors as a lack of engagement of the reward valuation network based upon a history of network inefficiency and low reward valuation of the targeted response, and that we would be discussing how this worked in the next few sessions. Melissa's communication skills, both internally and outwardly directed were pointed out. The impact from both of these perspectives was touched upon. Melissa was asked to complete the NCLT template in order to continue to refine the schema from which she was operating.

A Long Word About What We Just Said
The discussions we just described in brief are in fact a key feature of NCLT treatment. As such, some detail is warranted to have the practitioner understand why they happen. In specific, they happen because the NCLT practitioner wants to give the client a new schema (or framework) that will serve as a basis for the knowledge they will be acquiring that will guide the process of change. These discussions that provide the framework of this new schema formation are determined by client-based factors. Their complexity and intricacy depends on factors such as the developmental level and cognitive capacity of the individual to understand the material. In Melissa's case, the therapist had decided that Melissa understanding how her emotional responses, behaviors, impulse control, and decision-making processes were all connected. That they were not characterological flaws, but they were going to be a targeted part of the treatment and so wanted to provide an initial framework for the following sessions.

In discussing the interactions of the various schemas that comprise Melissa's response patterns, NCLT makes use of small world/rich world hub modeling of neurocognitive functioning. The literature regarding small world hub network models and their ability to describe neural networking models for impulsivity and decision making is complex. It will only be reviewed briefly here. Interested readers are directed to our earlier (Wasserman & Wasserman, 2016) work for a more detailed explanation.

The most important aspect of this literature for the current discussion is how NCLT views the development of issues in the areas deemed problematic for Melissa. Problems with poor choice making arise as a result of an interaction between constitutional factors such as the pace of myelination and basic neural networking structure, and related learning factors that determine the outcome of reward history. For example, there is clear evidence that ADHD represents a disorder of altered structural connectivity of the brain, characterized by distributed atypical white matter microstructure (Nagel et al., 2011). This same work demonstrates that later maturing frontolimbic pathways were abnormal in children with ADHD. This finding was considered due to delayed or decreased myelination. Overall, results were considered suggestive that early occurring (perhaps or likely prenatally) disruptions in white matter microstructure may play a key role in the early pathophysiology of ADHD.

In addition, literature demonstrates that individuals displaying issues with the regulation of impulses display both impaired executive control and enhanced reward sensitivities as compared to controls. How these two networks jointly interact to produce the valuation process and drive behaviors remains unclear (Dong, Lyn, Hu, Xie, & Du, 2015). Research suggests, however, that white matter micro architecture differences lead to impairments in executive control and inefficient inhibition of enhanced reward valuations. It has also been demonstrated that people with impulse control difficulties demonstrate impaired risk evaluation in general (Lyn, Zhou, Dong, & Du, 2015). In summary, this literature suggests that individuals with impulse control do not effectively create reward valuations that guide their choices. They either over emphasize certain aspects or features of the perceived reward, or fail to identify reward aspects at all.

How this comes about and the relationship of the contributing networks remains somewhat unclear at present, and different NCLT practitioners often choose to emphasize different aspects of the known information depending on the point they are trying to make, and their understanding of the client.

So these findings, delayed myelination, altered reward valuation and related risk assessment all contribute to the impulsive behavior associated with ADHD. We will leave aside the discussion about problems with one or the other potentially representing different disorders and go on to say that NCLT considers that the impulsive individual sitting before you represents the culmination of the interaction of these two networks. Disruptions of the white matter architecture due to delayed myelination means that these individuals have more difficulty bringing on network components related to both inhibition of undesirable responses and successful reward valuation that would drive more adaptive choices. This is because the unmyelinated neurons that comprise these networks are inefficient. Initially, that means that young children are driven to more intense stimuli. That is because the increased intensity is necessary to capture the attention of a more sluggish network. The more intense stimuli may be defined by others as more risky, explaining how those diagnosed with ADHD often find themselves in physical, financial, academic, and sometimes legal difficulties.

All of the above implies that individuals with attention problems really have difficult with reward valuation and related assignment of working memory (Wasserman & Wasserman, 2015), and depending on their age, may also still be displaying the effects of processing inefficiency related to delayed myelination. That is why what you emphasize is related to the nature of the individual sitting in front of you. For an adult who had had sufficient time for the myelination processes to be completed, delay does not mean never, it means it takes longer, so one would emphasize the reward valuation component stressing the necessity of reanalysis of stimuli valiances. On the other hand, if you were talking to a parent of a 3 year old, you would be emphasizing the processing inefficiency and need for intensity in choice selection. Simply stated, this is why behavior therapists insist on making the desired behavioral choice really, really rewarding, and why it frequently loses its effectiveness, or in our terms, reward valence.

Again, compounding the neurophysiological and resulting sequelae is Melissa's poor communication skills. Simply put, Melissa's processing styles, mirrored in her verbal communications, poses an issue with no resolution. The lack of completion irritates others who are looking for completion. It also has a very specific neuro-physiological impact on Melissa; the lack of completion speaks to the connectome and cortical connections specifically reaching the fronto-parietal lobe areas. These areas are associated with organization and decision making. There is research to suggest that in people diagnosed with ADHD, these areas are immaturely myelin-ated, and therefore not easily recruited. We posit that the ongoing practice of not making decisions and poor verbal completion of problem solving exacerbates or expands this neuropsychological process. That is, the lack of decision making has historically contributed to this process rather than exclusively caused it. It over-whelms Melissa with anxiety, and her poor integration results in her "shutting down." Correcting this lack of resolution became a primary goal of the therapist in order to assist the client in developing connections which would increase the likeli-hood of greater recruitment of decision making, planning, and organization related networks.

Homework: The Beginning of New Connectome Connections
In order to begin to intervene, Melissa was assigned the I Think–I Feel template. The assignment was to record, real or imagined, current or past examples of situa-tions, elaborating on how she felt and what she was thinking. Keeping in line with the NCLT model of practicing mental health, Melissa was instructed to remember that not all examples had to be problems. In fact, some positive examples were encouraged. After all, it was just as important for Melissa to learn how to share what she felt positive about with others as to express what she found problematic.

We have condensed quite a lot of material into these hypothetical first sessions. In actuality, much of what we were talking about was the explanation of the model which would occur quite automatically to a seasoned NCLT therapist. Melissa just had a discussion, some hypothesis testing and a brief explanation of the model. The complexity of the models was fleshed out of the ensuing sessions.

The Second Session
Based upon our initial discussion Melissa went home and asked her mother details about her early development and requested details on any issues she might have manifest. It turned out that Melissa's mother perceived Melissa as somewhat diffi-cult very early on. Melissa was an extremely finicky eater. She ate a very limited number of things and they had to be prepared the exact same way. This often meant that no matter what Melissa's mother planned on preparing for dinner, she had to prepare Melissa a separate dish. If Melissa's mother tried to get Melissa to eat what the family was eating, Melissa would try to taste it and break down crying. She complained that she hated how it tasted or smelled. This persisted well into Melissa's young adult life.

In addition, Melissa's mother clarified her school history. It turned out that Melissa had difficulty making it through the traditional school day. As it happened that Melissa was a very talented golfer, Melissa's mother decided to use this to their advantage and enroll her in the special curriculum offered with the dual sports program. This program allowed her to leave school early to play golf.

The acquisition of this information certainly helped confirm the clinician's hypotheses. It also had a remarkable effect on Melissa. Now Melissa was beginning to understand herself as something other than the identified problem in the family. She began to synthesize how all of these facets came together to produce someone who is not easily engaged, who is not terribly interested in traditional paths, why she is always the one who is most critical of the restaurant meals and atmosphere, and how others perceive her as moody and distant.

Melissa actually had some difficulty completing her template. She stated that she couldn't think of anything to write. We used the session to explore her week and translated events onto the template. Once Melissa saw how it helped clarify her thoughts, she felt encouraged and ready to apply this to her family interactions.

The Subsequent Sessions
Over the course of the next two or three sessions Melissa and the clinician continued to help Melissa clarify her issues and put them into complete thoughts. These complete thoughts were necessary so that Melissa could begin to recognize the major themes (schemas) that governed her thinking. She began to develop new response sets. Instead of shutting down, she placed increased effort on finishing her thoughts and making a plan to respond. Instead of being immediately overwhelmed, she was allowing herself more time to collect her thoughts before responding. She also began to think more about her choices and what possible positive and negative outcomes they might have. What is critical here is that Melissa was doing what humans are designed to do; she had identified a set of problems and was working on solutions to them. The problems were stripped of excess baggage and represented reasonable targets for her to focus on. None of this meant that there was anything wrong with her. To the contrary, all this meant is that she had learned to respond in a maladaptive fashion to certain things she found stressful and difficult, and recognizing that her chosen solutions were less than ideal she was engaged in developing a healthier health response pattern.

The next step was for her to apply her new skills in vivo. In fact, Melissa returned after these sessions and indicated that she was feeling much relieved. She stated that she was now better able to explain to her parents when she was getting neurophysiologically overwhelmed and needed to take a few minutes to organize her thoughts. She let them know that she would return to complete the conversation as soon as she had some clarity. She, nor they, now described her as sullen, moody, and selfish, but instead came to understand that the shutdown was neurophysiological, not personal.

Over the course of the next few sessions, Melissa also addressed her confusion about her career goals. The NCLT therapist was able to help her to understand that this was not an issue of Melissa intending to be selfish or "a bad person." Rather

Melissa came to understand that this was a constitutional issue: Melissa is not easily aroused neurophysiologically. She didn't love her profession, but chose it and was able to sustain herself through the program because she was intelligent and because her mother challenged her decision, in effect elevating her arousal and motivation. Once she actually got into the field, she lost interest. It lost its novelty. So did the city. Humans are attracted to novelty (Cohen, 2013). It is one of the key determinants of response gating. And so she left the city life to pursue something else. That of course lost its novelty as well. Now she is again bored and thinking about returning to her perception of the higher arousal inherent in a large city. Of course, it needs to be a city which also accommodates her hiking and rafting interests, hobbies with high arousal, and novelty values.

After several sessions Melissa indicated that she had not only clarified the issues that brought her to therapy but also developed a new set of response patterns that would help her continue to address these issues as they arose. Therapy was terminated.

You might ask, and what about Jeff? Was his selection and her dissatisfaction with him a reflection of the same general response schema we were working on? The short answer is, of course he was. Melissa was completely happy dealing with the issues that she had chosen; Jeff was for another day.

Melissa Returns

Melissa returned to therapy approximately 1 year later. She reported that she has followed up and continued to practice the skills she had learned in therapy. A return for additional sessions at some point is not an uncommon occurrence in NCLT treatment. After all NCLT is a learning-based model that requires practice and automation of new skills before additional training can be effective. This is true of any learning. New skills are continually appended to older pattern matched skills, and the development of a new group of responses proceeds in an incremental fashion. In fact, a client returning after some time likely speaks to their perception of the process as helpful and their being ready for the next step.

So, it is quite common that the client goes off to practice the new skills they have learned and does fairly well in general. After a while they run into something they can't puzzle out for themselves and come back in for a couple of sessions to see if they can develop an understanding of the schema that was driving their response to a new set of situations. Often, as we will see, these responses continue to be variations on a central theme.

Melissa now wants to talk about Jeff. Melissa has been dating Jeff for 5 years. They met in school. She describes him as a really nice guy and all of her friends seem to like him. He resides in the city she worked as an architect in, but now, since her move out of state, they travel to see each other. She, however, has reservations about the relationship. She is just not sure he is "the right one." Melissa is worried that there is something wrong with her. Even though she has reservations about Jeff, she is having a hard time letting go of him. She did not understand why she lacked the resolution to let him go even though at this point, she perceived Jeff as being the one who wanted out of the relationship. She wondered if this was yet another example of her indecision. Melissa asks you why, if she knows Jeff is not right for her, she gets excited about the possibility of seeing him when she goes back to the city.

Therapy, at this juncture, could have gone in so many directions. Therapy could have centered on Melissa's inability to commit. It could have focused on her lack of maturity in relationships. It could have focused on her fighting "acting like a grown up." It could have focused on her fears of letting go. NCLT predicts that the responses to these new sets of circumstances would be related to the core schemas that Melissa would have developed over time. We therefore chose to examine how the current set of issues related to the original schema regarding novelty and arousal. Specifically, Jeff was no longer novel. As he was no longer novel, he was no longer arousing and therefore the desire to pursue the relationship was diminished. In short, Melissa was once again bored, but this time it was with Jeff. Melissa confirmed, however, that Jeff seems to get interesting every time he is not available and her uncertainty regarding his desire to continue the relationship propels her to reengage. Jeff pulling away heightens Melissa's interest. It begins the dating challenge again and requires novel solutions to convince Jeff to come see her.

Melissa reports that she recognizes that she has never really been attracted to the physical Jeff. She was attracted to the perks that go along with being a couple—the friends, the social network, the promise of a future that contains important things for Melissa—being a wife and mother, for example. Although it is not entirely clear that being a wife and mother represented the next challenge for Melissa and that, having acquired them, she might tire of them as well. She believes, however, that she has internalized our society's values.

After some discussion, Melissa came to understand that Jeff represented something she found rewarding, but it was not *he* that was rewarding. The pattern of arousal that come with the "chase" was engaging. Alas, Jeff himself was not nearly engaging for her. Melissa came to understand that the pattern was the same whether it was a career, job, hobbies, or relationship; Novelty was arousing and engaged her.

Over the course of time none of these areas retained their novel and high reward valences. She would become disengaged by changing careers, hobbies, and partners. The question for Melissa was whether she could find someone who could sustain her interest over the long haul. It was pointed out that the onus could not be completely on the future partner; that no individual, however exciting, could sustain a unidirectional relationship. Melissa was encouraged to think about other aspects of the relationship that might sustain engagement after the novelty phase.

References

Carta, M., Balestrieri, M., Murru, A., & Hardoy, M. (2009). Adjustment disorder: Epidemiology, diagnosis and treatment. *Clinical Practice and Epidemiology in Mental Health, 5*, 15. doi:10.1186/1745-0179-5-15.

Cohen, R. (2013). Neuropsychology of attention: Synthesis. In R. Cohen (Ed.), *The neuropsychology of attention* (pp. 931–963). New York: Springer.

Connolly-Gibbons, M., Rothbard, A., Farris, K. W.-S., Thompsom, S., Scott, K., Heintz, L., et al. (2011). Changes in psychotherapy utilization among consumers of services for major depressive disorder in the community mental health system. *Administration and Policy in Mental Health and Mental Health Services Research, 38*(6), 495–303. doi:10.1007/s10488-011-0336-1.

Diagnostic and statistical manual of mental disorders. (2013). (5th ed.). Washington, DC: American Psychiatric Association.

Dong, G., Lyn, X., Hu, Y., Xie, C., & Du, X. (2015). Imbalanced functional link between executive control network and reward network explain the online-game seeking behaviors in internet gaming disorder. *Scientific Reports, 5*, 9197. doi:10.1038/srep09197. Retrieved from http://www.nature.com/articles/srep09197.

Grohol, J. (2009). *10 secrets your therapist won't tell you*. Retrieved from Psychcentral.com: http://psychcentral.com/blog/archives/2009/09/29/10-secrets-your-therapist-wont-tell-you/

Lyn, X., Zhou, H., Dong, G., & Du, X. (2015). *Progress in Neuro-Psychopharmacology and Biological Psychiatry, 56*(2), 142–148.

Nagel, B., Bathula, D., Hertling, M., Schmitt, D., Kroenke, C., Fair, S., et al. (2011). Altered white matter microstructure in children with attention-deficit/hyperactivity disorder. *Journal of the American Academy of Child & Adolescent Psychiatry, 50*(3), 283–292.

Osborne, S. (2015, June 20). *What do psychotherapists say about the importance, if any, of theory in their work with clients?* Retrieved from Roehampton University Research Repository (RURR): http://roehampton.openrepository.com/roehampton/handle/10142/618257

Wasserman, T., & Wasserman, L. (2015). The misnomer of attention deficit hyperactivity disorder. *Applied Neuropsychology: Child, 4*(2), 116–122. doi:10.1080/21622965.2015.1005487.

Wasserman, T., & Wasserman, L. (2016). *Depathologizing psychopathology*. New York: Springer.

Chapter 10
NCLT Clinical Procedures

As we have pointed out, depending on the stimuli and behavioral/emotional response targeted in treatment, NCLT practice can encompass a wide variety of clinical techniques. We have stressed that NCLT is an integrative model. As such, it can make use of many techniques, some of which are based on entirely different conceptual models. Recognizing the benefits of using the technique, even though conceptual differences exist between the models, is a strength of NCLT. NCLT practitioners can use a technique as long as they understand how the results and benefits they will obtain from its use will fit into the NCLT conceptual model. For example, if I want to teach a person to relax as one way to manage their stress-related physiological responses, I can use a meditation technique as long as the client and I understand how the benefits of that technique affect my physiologic response to stress.

This definition of an integrative model is different from the traditional understanding of integrative models. Those traditional models represent integrative therapy as a combined approach that brings together different elements of specific therapies because no single approach can encompass the totality of human psychological experience. Integrative models hold that each theoretical perspective describes an element of a person's psychological make up. NCLT is based upon a model of how people process and make use of the information they receive. It recognizes that a person can receive this information through many different kinds of experiences interacting with their connectome. NCLT also recognizes that these experiences have predictable impact on the psychological functioning of people, and it is these outcomes that we concern ourselves with in treatment.

The Third Wave

Hayes (2004) offered a view that indicated that behavior therapy could broadly be organized into three generations, or "waves," characterized by a "set or formulation of dominant assumptions, methods, and goals, some implicit, that help organize

© Springer International Publishing AG 2017

T. Wasserman, L.D. Wasserman, *Neurocognitive Learning Therapy: Theory and Practice*, DOI 10.1007/978-3-319-60849-5_10

research, theory, and practice" (p. 640). In response to a rebellion against the prevailing psychodynamic and gestalt traditions, the first wave of behavior therapy was hypothetically built upon the foundation of scientifically well-established basic principles. The applied technologies that derived from this foundation were designed to be well-operationalized and rigorously tested. These first treatments focused directly on problematic behavior and emotion, based on conditioning and neobehavioral principles. The goal would not be to resolve the hypothesized unconscious fears and desires of the clients. Rather the goal of treatment was targeted behavioral change.

The second wave began in the late 1960s when modern behavioral theoreticians began to recognize the limitations of treatments based upon simple associative concepts of learning, and turned to the use of more flexible mediational principles and mechanistic computer modeling. Cognition was added as a behaviorally defined target, and this in turn established a much more liberal and generous theoretical approach that included hypothesized internal psychological machinery. "Behavior therapists knew they needed to deal with thoughts and feelings in a more direct and central way. In the context of the failure of both associationism and behavior analysis to provide an adequate account of human language and cognition, the seeds planted by early cognitive mediational accounts of behavior change quickly flowered into the cognitive therapy movement" (p. 642). In the second wave, irrational thoughts, pathological cognitive schemas, or faulty information-processing styles were all targets for intervention. These could, and should, be weakened or eliminated through their detection, correction, testing, and disputation.

The third wave began when, as it should, science began questioning some of the assumptions of the second wave. In addition, questions arose concerning the limitations of the second wave interventions and the models of mental health that they are based upon. This third wave is characterized by a period of scientific intensity and creativity. This third wave was based upon a number of critical research findings. A shift in the understanding of the role of cognition in maladaptive behavior that indicated that rather than the form or frequency of specific problematic cognitions, focusing on the cognitive context and coping strategies related to these specific thoughts was important in successful treatment. In addition, more emphasis was placed on contacting the present moment redirecting treatment to the psychological context in which cognition occurs. In addition to these developments, Mindfulness-based cognitive therapy (Teasdale et al., 2002) provided clear demonstration that it was possible to alter the function of thoughts without first altering their form. Hayes (2004) provided a summary of third wave behavioral models that have developed in response to these developments. These models were "particularly sensitive to the context and functions of psychological phenomena, not just their form, and thus tend to emphasize contextual and experiential change strategies in addition to more direct and didactic ones. These treatments tend to seek the construction of broad, flexible, and effective repertoires over an eliminative approach to narrowly defined problems, and to emphasize the relevance of the issues they examine for clinicians as well as clients. The third wave reformulates and synthesizes previous generations of behavioral and cognitive therapy and carries them forward into questions, issues, and domains previously addressed primarily by other traditions, in hopes of improving both understanding and outcomes" (p. 658).

We will review Hayes' third wave model below. We believe that NCLT is just such a third wave model and that it meets the criteria for inclusion based upon that which was laid out above. Furthermore, we believe that NCLT can easily incorporate these models into a comprehensive treatment and theoretical rationale. What is different from these other models is that NCLT concerns itself with how the client learns, not just the client's reaction to a treatment intervention. As such, NCLT can easily incorporate other intervention systems. With recognition of this fact, there are certain procedures that are frequently used within NCLT and could arguably be said constitute the core of NCLT practice. What follows is a discussion of those procedures, the models that they are based upon, and a comparison of the particular models with NCLT theory.

Cognitive Behavioral Techniques

What Is Cognitive Behavior Therapy?

Since its inception as a short term, directed intervention for depression, cognitive behavioral therapy has expanded and produced a number of variants. Although the basic techniques and tenets of the approach are fairly straightforward, there are, as we have seen above, a plethora of specific treatments that can be categorized, more or less, as falling under the CBT model. These include cognitive therapy, problem-solving therapy, dialectical behavior therapy, meta-cognitive therapy, rational-emotive behavior therapy, cognitive processing therapy, mindfulness-based cognitive therapy, cognitive-behavioral analysis system of psychotherapy, and schema-focused therapy (Guadiano, 2008). It would be fairer to say that cognitive behavior therapy is a general classification of therapy, with a central tenet, rather than a single specific approach. It is now commonly utilized by many practitioners, and has a solid empirical basis regarding its efficacy (Butler, Chapman, Forman, & Beck, 2006). Despite the rich diversity, all cognitive behavioral techniques share a set of common elements.

CBT Is Based on the Idea That Cognitions Cause Feelings

Cognitive-behavioral therapy is based on the idea that thoughts cause feelings and resulting behaviors. External things like people, situations, and events are neutral, and our reactions to them are caused by our interpretations of them. By changing the way we think about things we can change the way we can think to feel/act better even if the situation does not change.

CBT Is Time-Limited

Cognitive-behavior therapy is considered among the most rapidly efficacious in terms of results obtained. The average is 16 sessions to completion, across all types of problems and approaches to CBT (National Association of Cognitive Behavioral Therapists, 2015). CBT tends to be more efficacious because it is directive, highly instructive, closed ended, and because of the fact that it makes use of home-based behavioral practice.

A Sound Therapeutic Relationship Is Necessary for Effective Therapy, but Is Not the Focus

As opposed to many forms of therapy which posit that people improve largely as a result of a positive therapeutic relationship, CBT therapists believe that people change because they learn how to think differently, and they practice and act on that learning.

CBT Is a Collaborative Effort Between the Therapist and the Client

Cognitive-behavior therapists strive to learn what their clients want out of life (their goals) and then help their clients achieve those goals. The therapist's role is to listen, teach, and encourage, while the client's role is to express and clarify their concerns. Clients are then asked to learn and implement that learning.

CBT Uses the Socratic Method

Cognitive-behavior therapists often ask questions designed to make cognitive and emotional concerns highly explicit. They also encourage their clients to ask questions and challenge themselves.

CBT Is Structured and Directive

Cognitive-behavioral therapists have a specific agenda for each session that is based on operationally defined goals and objectives. Specific techniques/concepts are taught during each session.

CBT Is Based on an Educational Model

CBT is based on the scientifically supported assumption that most emotional and behavioral reactions are learned. Therefore, the goal of therapy is to help clients unlearn their unwanted reactions and to learn a new way of reacting.

Treatment is based on a cognitive formulation of the beliefs and related behaviors that characterize a particular disorder. In addition, and very importantly for NCLT practice, treatment is also based on the recognition that there are individualized patterns of thoughts and behavioral responses based on patient experiences (Beck, 1995).

CBT/NCLT Similarities and Differences

The careful reader will note that many of these elements are characteristic of NCLT practice. In fact, an NCLT session looks very similar to some highly structured CBT procedures with respect to thoughts and feelings. There is, however, a major difference: NCLT recognizes that emotional responses can become automatized, and thereby arise without the benefit of cognitive effort, and without material being drawn into working memory.

Memory Reconsolidation

A key conceptual element at the core of NCLT practice is the research regarding memory reconsolidation which has been taken to demonstrate the concept of neural plasticity in response to treatment.

From the previous chapter we have identified the following steps, according to the memory reconsolidation model, for a maladaptive emotional memory and its related behavior to be modified. These steps regularly occur as part of NCLT practice.

1. Symptom identification. Actively clarify with the client what to regard as the presenting symptom(s). These include the specific behaviors, somatics, emotions, and/or thoughts that the client wants to eliminate and when they happen. This includes the percepts and contexts that evoke or intensify them.
2. Retrieval of target learning into explicit awareness, as a visceral emotional experience, the details of the emotional learning or schema underlying and driving the presenting symptom.
3. Identification of disconfirming knowledge. Identify a vivid experience (past or present) that can serve as living knowledge that is fundamentally incompatible with the model of reality in the target emotional learning retrieved in step 2, such that both cannot possibly be true. The disconfirming material may or may not be

appealing to the client as being more "positive" or preferred; what matters is that it be mutually exclusive with the target learning. It may be already part of the client's personal knowledge or may be created by a new experience.

There is a fourth step wherein the client verifies the new emotional response by generalizing it into new situations and contexts (Ecker, Ticic, & Hulley, 2013).

Coherence Therapy

These steps to memory reconsolidation feature prominently in coherence therapy (Bridges, 2016). Coherence therapy is a system of psychotherapy based in the theory that symptoms of mood, thought, and behavior are produced coherently according to the person's current mental models of reality, most of which are implicit and unconscious. As we have pointed out, NCLT advocates automaticity rather than unconscious, but that distinction does not prevent the use of coherence therapy techniques designed to alter patterns of memory connectivity from being utilized within an NCLT frame work. There are many similarities between the models. The basis of coherence therapy is the principle of symptom coherence. This principle holds that an individual's maladaptive behavior consisting of seemingly irrational, out-of-control symptoms are actually logical, cogent, orderly expressions of the person's self-constructed interpretations of the world rather than a disorder or pathology. Instead of the NCLT neurophysiologically based connectomics, coherence therapy refers to the brain–mind–body system. Emotional reaction is considered as an expression of logical (coherent) personalized schemas (constructs) which can include nonverbal, emotional, perceptual, and somatic elements, not just verbal-cognitive propositions. A therapy client's presenting symptoms are understood as an activation and enactment of specific schemas (constructs) (Ecker, Ticic & Hulley, 2012). The main activity of coherence therapy is the process of memory reconsolidation.

There are some basic steps to coherence therapy all of which can be utilized within an NCLT model. The main activity of coherence therapy is the use of experiential methods that create everyday awareness of how the maladaptive symptom is an active and meaningful facet of the client's existing solution to a specific problem of everyday life (Ecker & Hulley, 2002).

Focus on Coherence Therapy

The therapist begins by learning what the client identifies as the maladaptive behavior, thought or emotional pairings and what they want changed.

Discovery in Coherence Therapy

Once the problem is identified and operationalized, the therapist attempts to identify the full range of activities in which it occurs.

Integration in Coherence Therapy

The therapist helps the client isolate the maladaptive response so it can be recognized and worked on.

Real-Time Recognition

As in NCLT, to promote recognition and potential generalization of the new adaptive response, a coherence therapist would coach the client to recognize a symptom's occurrence between sessions. In addition, the NCLT therapist would also supply an adaptive response to be substituted in those same situations. This is handled differently in coherence therapy which posits that on occasion, that the mere recognition of the maladaptive symptomology's relationship to everyday behavior yields a positive transformation. When that does not occur, an additional step is required which involves prompting clients create a new, incompatible construct that disconfirms and dissolves the old one. The above is in no way a comprehensive summary of coherence therapy, and the interested reader is directed to the reference at the end of this chapter to gain a greater awareness of the model and its techniques.

Coherence therapy techniques are by no means the only way to produce the moment of disconfirmation required by memory reconsolidation. Understanding the requirements of memory reconsolidation, particularly the requirements of step 3, the identification of disconfirming knowledge, leads us to consider the frequent use of cognitive disputational techniques as part of NCLT practice.

A Word About Cognitive Disputation

Once considered the hallmark of effective cognitive behavior therapy there is recent evidence that cognitive disputation is not the active ingredient in the effectiveness of cognitive behavior therapy (Longmore & Worrel, 2007). This conclusion is based on three lines of converging research. Firstly, component analyses of treatment have failed to show that cognitive interventions provide significant added value to the therapy. Secondly, many cognitive behavioral treatments have achieved rapid symptomatic improvement prior to the introduction of specific cognitive interventions. Thirdly, there is a scarcity of data that changes in cognitive mediators are responsible for symptomatic change. NCLT makes use of cognitive disputational techniques in service of the larger goal to help the client understand that there are multiple ways of understanding an event, and that their current pattern of interpretation is the result of learning in interaction with environmentally mediated events. That is, NCLT goes beyond disputing a cognition. It challenges a schema.

A Case to Consider

Sara recently came into therapy. She reported a lifetime of depression and multiple suicide attempts. She wanted to address her feelings of anger toward her deceased mother. Sara explained that her mother had been a very competent professional who gave up her professional potential secondary to the demands of her unhappy marriage. She was fiercely independent and was intent on never imposing on others. Sara felt terrible upon learning that her mother had been unhappily married, but her mother professed it too late to do anything about. Sara remembers her as a very warm mother; Someone who literally cried with Sara when Sara got hurt. Sara vividly remembers watching television with her mother on many occasions. On one such occasion a character had committed suicide. Sara's mother declared it to have been his only option. Sara believed that this message was meant for her.

Sara's prior therapist correctly disputed the idea that her mother would want her to hurt herself. She encouraged Sara to talk to her mother about this. Sara asked her mother about this, who denied it, but Sara maintained "What else could she say?" Sara's schema of her relationship with her mother was just like everything else in Sara's perception of her mother's life; Sara was a disappointment to her. This made Sara characterologically flawed.

Following NCLT principles it was quickly ascertained that severe depression ran in the family. Therefore it was likely that Sarah herself has at least a predisposition to develop depressive disorder. We know that disputation had not worked to reduce the depression because Sarah had already dismissed the challenges. As a result of NCLT memory reconsolidation was achieved when Sara come to understand that although her mother was a warm and caring parent, she suffered from depression—the belief and consequential behaviors that she could have no impact on her own life and decisions. Her mother believed that suicide was a viable and indeed only option. Unfortunately, that was what she taught Sara, and that was what Sara learned. Sara also learned that in order to get affection, she had to be in distress. And so, Sara learned and practiced how to secure her mother's affection by hurting herself. It wasn't intentional on anyone's part. Nonetheless, Sara's mother never gave Sara the tools to fight the family genetics. Sara, who had internalized all of this as reflective of her own failings, now had a new schema. One where no one was to blame, but one wherein it was up to her, through therapy, to learn to be resilient.

Acceptance and Commitment Therapy (Hayes, 2004)

Acceptance and commitment therapy (ACT) emphasizes "psychological flexibility" and contextualism through mindfulness and the acceptance (as opposed to control) of distressing thoughts and feelings, while advocating using the personal goals and values of the clients as part of the process of changing behavior. Hayes has identified ACT as part of the "third Wave" of cognitive behavior therapies that are characterized by techniques that reduce or exclude direct cognitive disputation, relying instead on more indirect methods of addressing distorted cognition.

There are six core elements of ACT (Hayes, 2013) and we will review them here in relation to where they are consistent within an NCLT model. In general, the ACT technique is consistent to the NCLT model in that the client's responses are understood in the context of a naturally occurring experiential sequence. They are not to be directly challenged as inherently defective. Rather they are to be altered because the response set is maladaptive. NCLT will at times use cognitive disputation to challenge the conclusions of a specific strongly held belief system that is producing maladaptive behavior. However, the disputation is directed at altering the schema, and targets new behavioral responses rather than being satisfied with the altered cognition.

Acceptance

Acceptance is taught as an alternative to experiential avoidance and involves the active and aware embrace of those private events occasioned by one's history without unnecessary attempts to change their frequency or form, especially when doing so would cause psychological harm. For example, anxiety patients are taught to feel anxiety, as a feeling, fully and without defense. In NCLT, clients are taught that anxiety is a natural response to a variety of circumstances, some within a client's control, some not. As in ACT, for NCLT, acceptance (and defusion) is not the goal of treatment. Rather, it is a step towards altering a response pattern to produce more adaptive and desired responses.

Cognitive Defusion

In ACT, cognitive defusion is an activity designed to alter the undesirable functions of thoughts and related events, rather than trying to alter their form, frequency, or situational sensitivity. According to Hayes (2013) ACT attempts to change the way one interacts with or relates to thoughts by creating contexts in which their unhelpful functions are diminished. In NCLT terminology, changing adaptive responses and repairing adaptive responses to situations are the desirable activities. On some occasions, this implies altering an interpretation that is clearly idiosyncratic and maladaptive, and on others, it involves the client respecting their feelings and deciding to act differently in response to them.

As in NCLT, ACT recognizes numerous techniques that have been developed for a wide variety of clinical presentations. There are procedures that attempt to reduce the intensity of the maladaptive or disruptive thought, weakening the association between the thought and what it refers to ("I am worthless") or weakening the frequency of the thought in relation to a specific stimulus.

NCLT encourages people to accept that certain neurophysiological states will present/return, and to accept that they will present without intensifying (panicking) about the return. That is, oft times the NCLT therapist will cue the client that, e.g., anxiety will return, to expect it, and to nonetheless be able to remain in personal control.

Being Present

ACT promotes ongoing nonjudgmental contact with psychological and environmental events as they occur. NCLT advocates that clients see new psychological and environmental events as neutral. This paves the way for the client to see that responses already interpreted as threatening or anxiety producing are the result of experience and decision making. For both ACT and NCLT, the goal is to have clients experience the world more directly so that their reaction to it is more flexible. Both NCLT and ACT recognize the power of language to exert control over behavior; and encourage the use of language to observe and describe events, not to predict and judge them.

Self as Context

NCLT, ACT, and other therapeutic models take a life course perspective on the development of the concept of the self. This developmental interpretation holds that the understanding of "self" develops and enriches over a long period of time as a result of perspective taking interactions between the person and various environmental occurrences. NCLT therapists understand how this interaction affects the connectome, creating neurophysiological changes and resulting changes in the "self." For both models the "self" is implied, as opposed to being defined. As a result of the ever expanding interactions with the environment, the total self is unknowable and cannot be operationalized. In some sense this means that it is ever changing, or at least has the potential for change.

Values

Both NCLT and ACT consider values as important contributors to purposive action.

For NCLT, values represent complex verbally driven schema that stake out a pattern of decision making in relationship to environmental occurrences. The implications of these values/schemas can never be fully articulated by the client because they have not experienced every situation that might bring them into play. Values are viewed differently in ACT, which attempts to diminish the role of verbal processes that might lead to choices based on avoidance, social compliance, or rapid judgment.

Committed Action

Both ACT and NCLT focus on the development of larger and larger patterns of effective action linked to adaptive values. In terms of specific skill acquisition, both look very similar to traditional behavior therapy, and as a result, almost any empirically valid behavior change protocol can be adapted into either of the models. Features found in many behavioral treatment approaches are also found in ACT and NCLT. These features include therapy work and homework linked to short-, medium-, and long-term behavior change goals. Taken as a whole, each of these processes supports the other and targets psychological flexibility: the process of contacting the present moment fully as a conscious human being, and persisting in or changing behavior in the service of chosen values. The NCLT therapist understands that this process is not magical. It is the direct result of, and is directly resulting in, changes to the connectome. The NCLT therapist understands that by effecting and practicing change, the client is increasing the ability to make and then have access to healthier, more adaptive pathways.

Other Third Wave Methodologies and Models and Their Relationship to NCLT

Schema therapy (Young, Klosko, & Weishaar, 2003) was originally developed for the treatment of personality disorders. Schema therapy was derived from traditional cognitive therapy with and added emphasis on the concept of schemata and modes and the inclusion of other models of therapy. In this regard, it is similar to the constructionist components of NCLT. For example, for Schema therapy, a person's coping styles are behavioral responses to schemas. Maladaptive schemas are self-defeating emotional and cognitive patterns established from childhood and repeated throughout life. Maladaptive coping styles (such as overcompensation, avoidance, or abandonment) very often wind up reinforcing and expanding existing schemas comprised of maladaptive responses. Schema therapy comprises a large spectrum of techniques to address emotions, cognitions, and behavior in the present life of the patient, within therapy and related to events and experiences in the past. Schema therapy is integrative in the sense that it uses emotion activation techniques originating in Gestalt and Psychoanalytic techniques yet, it is strictly behavioral in the models communicated to the patient. One of the dominant skills trained in schema therapy is to recognize the present dysfunctional modes of functioning, and to have that behavior guided by a healthy adult model.

Dialectical Behavior Therapy (Linehan & Koerner, 2012)

Dialectical behavior therapy (DBT) assumes that skills deficits in the area of emotion regulation are at the center of many disorder of mental health. As a result, DBT practitioners teach a broad spectrum of skills in the areas of mindfulness, distress tolerance, emotion regulation, and interpersonal effectiveness. DBT theory posits that some people are prone to react in a more intense and out-of-the-ordinary manner toward certain specific emotional situations, primarily those found in interpersonal relationships (romantic, family, and friend). DBT theory suggests that some people's arousal levels in such situations can increase far more quickly than is desirable, reach a higher level of emotional stimulation, and take a significantly greater amount of time to return to baseline arousal levels. All of these concepts are in sync with the NCLT model of arousal and maintenance of aroused states (Wasserman & Wasserman, 2016) and as a result, DBT treatment approaches can easily be fit into an NCLT model.

The Fourth Wave?

Given its ability to integrate most therapeutic models within its conceptual framework, it might be possible to describe NCLT as the beginning of a fourth wave. These would be models that were able to describe the multiplicity of factors that contribute to the development of mental functioning in people, while including the ever increasing contributions of neuroscience. In addition, these models have the potential to incorporate and explain all intervention techniques under one coherent framework. This wave will have the capacity to not only conceptualize a case presentation and apply interventions, but also conceptualize a case presentation from a contextual and life course model, apply interventions specifically targeting particular schemas, and be able to teach the principles underlying both maintaining the presentation of the issues and how to impact their resolution. This wave integrates psychology and neuroscience, producing an empirically validatable and validated theory and therapy.

References

Beck, J. (1995). *Cognitive behavior therapy*. New York/London: Guilford Press.

Bridges, S. (2016). Coherence therapy: The roots of problems and the transformation of old solutions. In H. Tinsley, S. Lease, & N. Wiersma (Eds.), *Contemporary theory and practice in counseling and psychotherapy* (pp. 353–380). Los Angeles: Sage Publications. ISBN: 9781452286518. OCLC 894301742.

Butler, A., Chapman, J., Forman, E., & Beck, A. (2006). The empirical status of cognitive-behavioral therapy: A review of meta-analyses. *Clinical Psychology Review, 26*(1), 17–31. doi:10.1016/j.cpr.2005.07.003.

Ecker, B., & Hulley, L. (2002). Deep from the start: Profound change in brief therapy is a real possibility. *Psychotherapy Networker, 26*(1), 64, 46–51.

Ecker, B., Ticic, R., & Hulley, L. (2012). *Unlocking the emotional brain eliminating symptoms at their roots using memory reconsolidation*. East Sussex, UK: Routledge.

Ecker, B., Ticic, R., & Hulley, L. (2013). A primer on memory reconsolidation and its psychotherapeutic use as a core process of profound change. *Neuropsychotherapist, 1*, 82–88. doi:10.12744/tnpt(1)082-099.

Guadiano, B. (2008). Cognitive-behavioral therapies: Achievements and challenges. *Evidenced Based Mental Health, 11*(1), 5–7. doi:10.1136/ebmh.11.1.5.

Hayes, S. (2004). Acceptance and commitment therapy, relational frame theory, and the third wave of behavioral and cognitive therapies. *Behavior Therapy, 35*, 639–665.

Hayes, S. (2013, July 23). *The six core processes of ACT*. Retrieved from Association for Contextual Behavioral Science: https://contextualscience.org/the_six_core_processes_of_act

Linehan, M. M., & Koerner, K. (2012). *Doing dialectical behavior therapy*. New York: Guilford Press.

Longmore, R., & Worrel, M. (2007). Do we need to challenge thoughts in cognitive behavior therapy? *Clinical Psychology Review, 27*(2), 173–187. doi:10.1016/j.cpr.2006.08.001.

National Association of Cognitive Behavioral Therapists. (2015). *Cognitive-behavioral therapy*. Retrieved from National Association of Cognitive Behavioral Therapists: http://www.nacbt.org/whatiscbt.htm

Teasdale, J. D., Moore, R. G., Hayhurst, H., Pope, M., Williams, S., & Segal, Z. V. (2002). Metacognitive awareness and prevention of relapse in depression: Empirical evidence. *Journal of Consulting and Clinical Psychology, 70*, 275–287.

Wasserman, T., & Wasserman, L. (2016). *Depathologizing psychopathology*. New York: Springer.

Young, J., Klosko, J., & Weishaar, M. (2003). *Schema therapy: A practitioner's guide*. New York: Guilford Press.

Chapter 11
Parables and Paradigms

Parables are frequently used in many forms of therapy (Pancner, 1978; Warnock, 1989). A parable is a tale, or story, that sets the familiar in a nonfamiliar context where the meaning is derived from the story itself. It does not directly teach the meaning. The meaning is abstracted from the interpretation of the story provided by either the listener, or the teller (Morris, 1969). Therapists use parables, stories, and examples in many different ways. NCLT uses them to assist learning and provide practice samples. Rather than challenge the presenting issue directly, which can often lead to the client defending their position, clients often find it easier to apply new meaning to emotionally neutral material before they apply it to the emotionally laden material that brought them to treatment. Parables often contain an element of humor which also serves to engage the clients in the learning process.

Why Stories Are Important

There are reasons why stories are successfully incorporated in many psychotherapy practices. It is because they work with how the brain is programmed to learn and retain information. Your brain is programmed to recognize patterns of information. In fact, one of the initial steps in learning is, after the identification of the new information, the classification of that new material within existing patterns of information. As we shall soon see, stories provide an important way of scaffolding new information around newly created schemes. That is because stories are also recognizable patterns, and we use them to find meaning in the world around us. When we tell a story or remember a story, we find ourselves in them. Our stories are personal to us (Jones, 2014). Stories also have some unique features that support learning. For example, when a person hears a story, their brain not only processes the language, but initiates network functions that would activate if you were actually in the story yourself (Feldman, 2008). We have all had experiences wherein we have cried during a movie or related parts of a book to others, because they resonate with us.

© Springer International Publishing AG 2017
T. Wasserman, L.D. Wasserman, *Neurocognitive Learning Therapy: Theory and Practice*, DOI 10.1007/978-3-319-60849-5_11

They create emotional arousal. In addition, the brain doesn't just stop at adding experiences. When listening to meaningful stories, your brain makes associations and connections with other related material, the result of which is that you develop thoughts, opinions, and ideas that align with the person telling the story (Eagleman, 2015). Telling stories supports and enriches the therapeutic relationship. So when you tell a story that has influenced your own thinking, you can actually influence the thinking of your client.

We are going to discuss some of our favorite therapeutic parables and examples, and talk about when we use them, and why.

Introducing a Patient to NCLT

There are probably as many ways to start the process of therapy as there are clinicians. Since NCLT favors instructive techniques, we have found that it is often good to begin therapy with a guide to how the process will unfold. In order to accomplish this, we sometimes use scenarios, and the parable of the bear in the woods is one such example. We are of course mindful that if we want psychological movement, it needs to be presented from someone with whom the patient can relate. So besides being as personable as possible, we provide a thumbnail sketch of ourselves and our orientation.

After brief introductions and the "general housekeeping" of starting a new patient, we would begin to introduce the theoretical underpinnings of NCLT to our clients in a very succinct and easily understandable way. We might explain that NCLT is a therapeutic strategy that respects the integration of the brain–body relationship; that the brain and mind are one, and that the brain and body is an integrated unit. We stress that NCLT sees the person as a whole. We explain that NCLT looks at what brings a person into therapy with a healthy respect for that person's individual psychological history and neurophysiology. We explain that we are going to be working on helping that person understand the etiology of these issues wherever possible, how we maintain them (automaticity), the neurophysiological, behavioral and emotional sequelae, and how they have generalized. We always include the idea that we are going to work on developing new skills to help that person deal with whatever is going on in a way that reduces their symptoms. We, as the clinician/scientists, know that the neurophysiological patterns have been created. So, as we touched upon previously, we never promise to make their particular symptomology go away. Rather, we assure our clients that we will work together to make the symptomology less intense, present less frequently and be of a shorter duration, because they will be gaining new skills which will eventually, with practice, replace the old connections; that is, alter the cognitive and emotional response sets.

Therapy is about learning, to learn new and adaptive ways of dealing with the problems one has identified. Research is clear that in order to learn effectively, we need a scaffold upon which to attach our new information, and we need to make the new information notable, relevant, and not too discrepant from that of the person's presenting position in order for it to be accepted and incorporated. Therefore, we want to present a scaffold upon which we can hang the new information we are going to impart.

The Bear in the Woods Scenario

Remember, NCLT uses strategies and techniques specific to the client and their presenting needs. The "Bear in the Woods Paradigm" provides a template which can be tailored through both the clinician's application, and the client's responses. It is a blank canvas onto which the patient can map their responses. What they say, how they say it, and what they emphasize, tells us a lot about how they processes, and the systematic way in which they relate to their environments. In other words, it gives us some initial information about the general primacy of a person's response set, their automatic response sets and schemas. The Bear in the Woods example produces a tremendous amount of information for us as clinician. Information which needs to be verified through further clinical observation and interaction, but nonetheless, information which provides a good beginning hypothesis as to how this person responds and processes.

The scenario follows:

Let's pretend that you and I are walking through the woods. It is a bright and sunny day and we are enjoying our conversation and not necessarily concentrating on what is going on around us. We are on a trail, and ahead of us is a large rock outcropping that the trail winds around, but obscures our view of what's ahead. We walk around the rock and suddenly, in the middle of the trail, you see a large brown bear. What is worse, the bear is pretty close, and if we continue moving it will definitely see us. What would you feel? What would you think? What would you do? Some answers could include the following:

John's response: "That's it. I'm lunch."
Sally's response: "Terrified."
Bill's response "Finally."
Mark's response "Cool."

Please tell me about your response. Tell me about what you think, how you feel and what you might do.

Introducing NCLT Principles

After obtaining their response, we would go on to point out that these responses are unique to them, that the scenario is neutral as regards responses, and how they respond is determined by an interplay of inborn flight or fight responses and previous learning experiences. They are usually skeptical, but this provides a perfect opportunity to challenge the idea that responses are fixed. In keeping with the NCLT approach to active participation, we ask directed questions such as: What would John likely think if he never saw a bear, and only read about them in stories where people got eaten by them? What would Sally likely feel never having been so close to a bear? And now we might challenge the preconception that all is lost: What would make Bill say "Finally" or Mark say "Cool"? What if Bill has had recently received a grant to study this particular type of bear? What if Mark had being able to observe this particular type of bear on his bucket list of things to do? We would also go on to explain that while the initial response would be predetermined by prior experiences or beliefs, it would not have to stay that way. New experiences and related learning could produce new responses. You may even decide to go on to study zoology!

Now that we have the client's attention, we are going to continue to expand upon these constructs. Namely, we are going to state the principle that they just helped us establish: that emotions and or cognitions are purely the result of our interpretations, and that these interpretations and resulting states are unique to each of us. Remembering that people will discount information that is too discordant to them, we might use the bear as an example because, although it is emotionally arousing, it is less emotionally laden than one that is personal to the client. We want them to be engaged, but more emotionally neutral so that they can better assimilate new information. We have found that using a nonemotionally laden exemplar allows the client to learn the necessary material without having to deal with a subject that in the past may have been too difficult to deal with. We say "necessary material" because as we stated earlier, the bear paradigm is a template. It will be used later on in therapy as well.

Using the Bear in the Woods Scenario to Begin the Therapeutic Discussion

Emotional Primacy

As we indicated above, it is important to pay attention to how a person responded to your questions. That is, did they respond with a feeling or with a cognition. In NCLT recognizing the importance of a therapeutic relationship, we also recognize the importance of "speaking the same language" as our client's. That is, we try to establish their primary primacy response type, and speak to that. Let us assume that the current primacy response type is emotional ("I'm terrified!").

Using the scenario above, we would point out that there were many possible potential reasons for feeling terrified, as well as many reasons to not be terrified at all. For example, in response to seeing the bear, and receiving an answer indicating fear, we would suggest that the fear is based upon the belief that "He's going to eat me". We would then go on to present a number of scenarios which would universally result in alternative *emotional* states. For example, we would ask how that person would feel if they came all the way to these woods specifically to see these bears. That person might feel happy, or delighted. How would that person feel if they had secured a grant to study these bears and got to see one on their first day in the area. Under that circumstance, one might feel delighted or excited. We might ask "What if you had done your research and knew that these bears tend to be docile unless threatened". We would respond that then you might feel wary, but under emotional control. We want our client to understand that emotions are not fixed, they exist on a continuum, and that responses represent a choice.

Cognitive Primacy

The same scenario can be used when attempting to address a person tending toward cognitive primacy. We might present that under the same conditions, the cognitive responder might chose to *think* that he is lucky to have seen the one animal he was particularly interested in. Or that now he will be able to pursue his grant. Or that he knows these bears are generally docile, and so as long as he keeps his distance and doesn't make any sudden moves, he is fine. Cognitions are not fixed. For the purposes of intervention, we need to understand that past interpretation influences current interpretation. Therapy is about guided assistance to making new attributions to learned and often generalized associations. In order to best accomplish that goal, we again want to work within the processing style, or framework of the client.

Why a Bear in the Woods?

This scenario allows us to help explain to people the effects of their prior learning and their response sets or schemas. It also allows us to "depathologize" the response set by explaining it from a neurophysiological and learning perspective, rather than focusing on the person's maladaptive or perceived inadequacies. The bear paradigm allows us to explain the flight or fight response. It allows us to explain how the initial response may have been very adaptive, but that it is designed to be a short-term response. Our brain/body is supposed to return to homeostasis. But what if we have (lifelong?) long-term practice becoming this neurophysiologically aroused? We explain that this results in a hypersensitivity to becoming anxious/fearful/stressed, etc. We are now accomplishing two things; we are teaching the client how they became this way from a non-characterological perspective, and we are teaching them how this response is being maintained.

Remember that people tend to categorize information. That renders it not novel. We want an image or a phrase that will get someone's attention and act as a shorthand for the new information we are imparting. Often times a client will look to us for an explanation of, e.g., why they were so anxious the past few days under certain circumstances. Although the therapist will initially likely have to prompt the explanation, the explanation will be incorporated. It is engaging, explanatory, and not too threatening. This increases the likelihood that, within a very short period of therapeutic time, the client will come up with the answer "The bear in the woods." It allows them to step away from their own experience and incorporate the principle.

John and the Bear

John has been in therapy for approximately a year. John came in angry at the world. If there was one thing John was initially proud of about himself, it was that he would "go nuclear" on someone if they tried to bully him. True to NCLT, we examined John's history, including his developmental and medical history. This revealed that John had a chronic medical condition which had affected his growth. He had a hard time in school as he was frequently sick. He had few friends because of bullying because of his size. John worked long and hard on understanding his easily triggered aggression. The "bear in the woods" parable was invaluable to the therapeutic process. It allowed us to talk about how John developed his defensive posture without therapy "attacking" John for his response style. It allowed John to give voice to feeling bullied by the bigger boys who also socially rejected him. It helped John understand that, of course, he would always be wary, he had a long history of being teased and bullied as a teen. This also helped explain how John became anxious. While anticipating being bullied made sense as a teen, it was now maladaptive. Through therapy, and through the use of this parable, John was able to easily understand why any criticism was now perceived as a threat. When he offered examples, he was easily able to explain his own behavior using the encounter as similar to one if he were to encounter "a bear in the woods." He came to understand how he came to "expect" to encounter a bear in the woods, and how his brain/body reacted accordingly with a fight or flight response. As John learned to control his aggressive responding, therapy turned to his anxiety. Treating his anxiety utilized a multipronged approach. In keeping with our current parable, let us look at how John maintained his own anxiety: John was employed in a setting that required him to work as part of a team. If he was too slow or made a mistake, the product was held up. John came in and stated that he had panicked at work. Through clarification of his thoughts, John was able to share that he perceived himself as being at a shooting range, with he himself as the target. Returning to our bear in the woods parable, John was able to see how responding physiologically to the threat of a bear attacking and his recent experience would both induce panic. By addressing how to handle ourselves if we did encounter the bear, John was better able to transfer the same principles to his own situation.

A Sample Worksheet for the Bear in the Woods

Below is a worksheet to help your clients ascertain what it is that they are feeling, and subsequently thinking, that is maintaining their distress. Note that the sentence stem begins with a request to determine how they are feeling. Options are presented because, as we have stated, often times clients confuse feelings and thoughts. Providing the list also minimizes the likelihood of a client being ambiguous about how they feel. Also note the use of the "I" pronoun. The "I" pronoun is critical. It is critical because the tendency of people is to tell us how they feel because of what someone *else* did or something that happened *to them*. This "I" "forces" the client to begin to speak about themselves—their feelings, their thoughts.

The Bear in the Woods Worksheet

Let's pretend that you and I are walking through the woods. It is a bright and sunny day and we are enjoying our conversation and not necessarily concentrating on what is going on around us. We are on a trail and ahead of us is a large rock outcropping that the trail winds around but our view of what's ahead is obscured. We walk around the rock and suddenly, in the trail, you see a large brown bear. Some answers could include the following:

John's response: "That's it. I'm lunch".
Sally's response: "Terrified."
Bill's response "Finally".
Mark's response "Cool".

After hearing the scenario please pick out your response from amongst the following possibilities. We have left a space to fill in another word that best describes your anticipated emotional response.

Worksheet—Emotive			
Sad	Angry	Worried	Apprehensive
Calm	Happy	Scared	Annoyed
Irritated	Elated	Wary	Anxious
Joyful	Furious	Devastated	Appreciative
Terrified	Ashamed	Embarrassed	Guilty

_____

Please describe what you might be thinking about

_____
_____
_____
_____
_____

Please complete the following sentences. Pick the sequence you feel would be most comfortable for you

I Feel _____

Because I think that

<u>I</u> _____

Or the following Worksheet—Cognitive

I think that I _____

And so I feel _____

Using the Template Later On in Therapy

Please note that the I feel/I think and emotional response options can be used all by themselves. This template version proves to be a very helpful tool in getting clients to clarify their issues, feelings, and maintaining belief sets. It also forces them, again, to speak about themselves, an imperative for therapeutic progress. Lastly, by assigning it as a homework exercise, it means the client is practicing. By directing the client to complete the template, it requires consideration of each point or issue. That provides the therapist with the ability to address each point or issue without becoming overwhelmed by the conglomeration of feelings and thought and examples a client may initially present. Although the initial material may not be consistent with our ultimate goals, it provides us with ongoing feedback about which schemas remained important during the week and what response the client had to them. As therapy progresses, we have the client's self-correct their worksheets. It is a perfect venue for providing the client with a problem solving approach to what is bothering them, their perspective and ultimately, how they can address it. The "take home" worksheet would simply be five templates of

I feel _____ because I think that I _____.

A typical initial example might be " I feel sad because I think he is being mean." This type of response is very rich in therapeutic material. Things to be addressed may include the fact that thinking one is being mean implies a deliberate emotional intent on their part. Perhaps this needs to be revisited. Another area to be addressed may be why this client responds to someone being mean with sadness?

A sound example might be "I feel angry because I think that I am being taken advantage of." This feeling state is now consistent with the client's beliefs. This now directs the therapist to helping the client ascribe adaptive emotional responses to situations, or to teach assertive training skills, or improve communications skills. In any event, it is a path to appropriate therapeutic intervention.

Therapy Parables

There are several key principles of therapy that routinely get discussed and we have developed several parables that help therapists introduce these principles/topics to their clients.

A Parable for the Principle That You Can't Please Everyone

The principle that you can't please everyone is firmly rooted in the cognitive behavioral literature, and is found in the literature of many other disciplines including psychoanalysis (Charatan, 2015). NCLT has a rather traditional cognitive behavior take on that, and points out that in most circumstances, it is quite impossible to achieve a persona that would in fact please everyone with everything one does. In addition to the cognitive disputation of the idea, an NCLT practitioner would also focus on the learned and automated emotional responses that would accompany the cognition when a person failed to meet that lofty expectation.

Here is a rather therapeutically famous fable by Aesop that is used to teach this principle. It has been adapted many times and appears in many places in many versions.

The Man, the Boy, and the Donkey (Jacobs, 1914)

A man and his son were once going with their Donkey to market. As they were walking along by its side a countryman passed them and said: "You fools, what is a Donkey for but to ride upon?"

So the Man put the Boy on the Donkey and they went on their way. But soon they passed a group of men, one of whom said: "See that lazy youngster; he lets his father walk while he rides."

So the Man ordered his boy to get off, and got on himself. But they hadn't gone far when they passed two women, one of whom said to the other: "Shame on that lazy lout to let his poor little son trudge along."

Well, the man didn't know what to do, but at last he took his boy up before him on the Donkey. By this time they had come to the town, and the passers-by began to jeer and point at them. The man stopped and asked what they were scoffing at. The men said: "Aren't you ashamed of yourself for overloading that poor Donkey of yours—you and your hulking son?"

The Man and Boy got off and tried to think what to do. They thought and they thought, till at last they cut down a pole, tied the Donkey's feet to it, and raised the pole and the Donkey to their shoulders. They went along amid the laughter of all who met them till they came to Market Bridge, when the Donkey, getting one of his feet loose, kicked out and caused the boy to drop his end of the pole. In the struggle the Donkey fell over the bridge, and his fore-feet being tied together he was drowned.

"That will teach you," said an old man who had followed them "Please all, and you will please none".

The Principle That You Can't Please Everyone So You Might As Well Please Yourself

Suppose you entered a beauty and talent pageant that ran over several weeks and involved a series of judging opportunities with the same judges. On the first opportunity nine of the ten judges vote for you and one votes for someone else.

You are excited, but based upon the principle that one can always improve, you ask the judge who did not vote for you what you could have done to earn their vote.

"No offense" says the judge, "I really liked you, I just prefer blondes."

As you are a brunette you will never get that judges vote so you decide to do something about it and so you go out and dye your hair blonde. Confident now, you go out and enter phase two of the contest, and sure enough the judge who likes blondes votes for you. However, this time you only get eight votes. Perplexed you approach the two judges who voted for you last week but not this week and ask them why they switched their vote. No offense, they both say, but we prefer natural color.

Determining that nine votes are better than eight you go out and change your hair color back to its original for the last phase of the contest. After the votes are counted, you now receive only six votes. Perplexed, you approach the judges who now have not voted for you. Besides the one who likes blonds, the other three answer "Because we don't like people who change their minds so frequently."

Teaching the Principle of Probabilistic Reward Valuation

Teaching concepts around probabilistic reward valuation, the process by which we calculate the probability and benefits of a prospective outcome, is one of the foundational activities in NLT. The process by which people make predictions about the affective nature of their environments, and to their ability to exert control over the choices that they make, is one of the most important skills that people learn in NCLT. For all people, maximizing perceived rewards and minimalizing perceived threats to homeostasis are critical to both happiness and longevity. Decision theory is a formal framework that allows us to describe and pose quantitative questions about optimal and approximately optimal behavior in such environments (Dayan & Daw, 2008).

While a discussion of probabilistic reward theory and the related signal detection theory is beyond the scope of this book, suffice it to say that there is substantial literature that individuals are sophisticated signal detectors and deciders based upon their ability to determine the reward-punishment ratio of the various choices that they have to make (Stocker & Simoncelli, 2006). People make thousands of decisions every day. Many of these represent situations that are encountered so often, that the responses become automated. Human behavior is remarkably sensitive to, and responsive to, alterations in the payoffs for different options. NCLT uses these theories to teach the idea that people are constantly making choices based on reward valuation, and therefore choices represent options, as opposed to fact. While so many of our everyday choices are automated, the automatization represents choices made on the basis of a consistent reward valuation. Once established in working memory, these valuations can be examined, and if necessary changed.

People have problems with this construct in the abstract despite the fact that they recognize, that it is obvious, to most people, that they will select the most preferred choice. Still, most people have problems with how ubiquitous this operation is in everyday life. This scenario appears to help them get the message:

Let's suppose you have just sat down to dinner and your plate has four items on it: A piece of chicken, some carrots, rice, and some stuffing. You are holding your fork over the plate. What determines what you pick first, or how do you choose what to eat?

Most people when first asked this question looked at you in a rather perplexed manner as they have never thought about how this process occurs (because it is so automatic). After some questions, they come around to the idea that they pick the thing they like the most, or in some cases eat the thing they like the least. In either event, it is easy to move to talking about the fact that they are making decisions all the time based on their internal calculations and that, if they want to make different choices they have to recalculate and reattribute the rewards and negatives assigned to each potential choice.

The Fact That Words Do Not Have the Power to Hurt You. It Is What You Decide About the Words Being Said That Hurts You

This is another idea that receives rather broad support from a variety of therapeutic disciplines. The NCLT interpretation is similar to the cognitive behavioral model that asserts that words are inherently neutral and achieve their power as a result of the perception and associations of the person who hears them. The following is often used when trying to demonstrate this concept to a client:

Suppose you are walking down the street, and as you approach the corner, you hear a person saying some terrible things to passersby. This person, who is very shabbily dressed and clearly in need of a bath, is questioning the parentage of each individual that walks by, and implying that the current target of the invective is in league with the Martians who have landed and are taking over the mind of people in the city where you live. You reach the corner and it becomes your turn. Apparently, one of your parents was a member of an alien species and you yourself are a Martian in disguise. How would you feel?

Most, if not all people, readily answer that the words mean nothing and that they would ignore the person and continue on their way without a second thought. The therapist follows this admission with the question: Then how would the same words coming from (Fill in the name of the person they were upset about) be any different? Most people acknowledge that it was not necessarily the words themselves that hurt, but that knowing that this same person mentioned above was upset with them, would upset them. That is, the words came from someone they value. That allows the discussion to move to the value of the perception of others, and the fact that you can't always please everyone.

The Wisdom of Practicing Something Before You Are in a Stressful Situation Having to Implement It

Stress in this context means a level of arousal and discomfort that is disturbing to the individual. NCLT recognizes that a mild degree of tension and arousal must exist between what is being learned and what is already known in order for the new learning or one's performance to be effective.

The literature on the deleterious effects of excessive stress indicates that learning is impaired when a person is too stressed (Kuhlmann, Piel, & Wolf, 2005). Remember, for NCLT, stress is the negative emotional interpretation of a physiological state. Just as with the interpretation of words, the interpretation of arousal is subjective, and the emotional response exists on a continuum. More specifically, there is growing research evidence that indicates that stress, either before or after learning, influences memory and impairs retention of information being processed when the individual is under stress (Schwabe & Wolf, 2010). That in turn affects performance. We recognize that from our own histories. Think about when you had a test coming up. If you experienced no arousal, you likely did poorly because of a lack of sufficient arousal. If you had too much arousal, or stress, you likely did poorly as well. Since NCLT is a learning-based model NCLT practitioners encourage their clients to learn new material under optimal conditions and in relatively stress-free situations. This may not always be possible or practical as many of the individuals we see are under almost constant stress or on occasion, if they are a child, out of control. Nonetheless, there must be times when the person is under less physiological stress. That is when we want our clients to practice as it leads to more efficient learning.

The example below is one that is used with teenagers as well as adults. It is used to encourage people to practice a new skill before the actually have to use it. We therefore encourage the client to learn what to do when they see a trigger that they have been taught will typically lead them to a stress-filled situation before they encounter the trigger. We introduce this concept by using the following example which seems to have a high attention getting value for teens and adults alike;

We ask "Do you drive a stick shift car?" Likely, driving a stick shift vehicle is exciting to teens and so you have now captured their attention. Adults are either nostalgic or confess they never learned to drive a stick. Therefore, almost always these days, the answer is no. Once they verify that they cannot drive a stick shift, we go on to describe the following scenario and ask a question (questions engage people). We say "Suppose you and your friends were going to rob a bank and you were the getaway driver. The only car you have is a stick shift. Do you think that the best time to learn would be while you were sitting outside the bank waiting for your fellow robbers to get into the getaway car?" Of course, they always agree that would be foolish. You then go on to ask how much practice you would need to have and when the best time to practice would be. The answers become self-evident; under a low stress situation and until I became proficient.

This example is also excellent for the client who comes to session and tells you that they did not do their practice homework because nothing bad happened that week. You would use the above example to demonstrate to them why that in fact was the perfect week to be practicing.

Many parents come to our office with children who tantrum frequently. It is routine for them to ask what they can do to stop the tantrum once it has begun. In these situations it is routine for us to say that nothing can be done at that point. The very nature of a tantrum is because of the magnitude of arousal leading to a loss of control. A person in a tantrum is no longer in control of themselves, and clearly incapable of engaging in any activity that would immediately serve to reregulate themselves. The correct intervention is again, identifying a trigger and having the child practice the adaptive response when the child is not stressed. Practice will enable the younger child to become more proficient in the more adaptive behavior, and more readily engage it (likely initially needing prompts secondary to poorer generalization in younger children) when presented with triggers. For them, we offer the suggestion to "play a game" wherein the parent is going to deliberately say something they know is generally a trigger. Depending on the developmental level of the child, this may be telling them you have changed your mind about something, you are going to be making their least favorite food for dinner, etc. You let them know in advance that this is coming, again, depending on the developmental level of the child, within a given timeframe. If the child can hear the typical stressor and respond appropriately, they get reinforced. We would also teach the adult client how "practicing" behavior becomes a default setting. So we can either have the child practicing tantrumming or socially appropriate responding.

References

Charatan, D. (2015, April 24). *How trying to make everyone happy can make you miserable.* Retrieved from Psychology Today: https://www.psychologytoday.com/blog/meaningful-you/201504/how-trying-make-everyone-happy-can-make-you-miserable

Dayan, P., & Daw, N. (2008). Decision theory, reinforcement learning. *Cognitive, Affective, & Behavioral Neuroscience, 8*(4), 429–453. doi:10.3758/CABN.8.4.42.

Eagleman, D. (2015). *The brain: The story of you.* New York: Random House.

Feldman, J. (2008). *From molecule to metaphor: A neural theory of language.* Cambridge: MIT Press.

Jacobs, J. (1914). *Aesop's fables.* New York: P.F. Collier and Son's.

Jones, S. (2014, April 24). *The psychology of stories: The storytelling formula our brains crave*. Retrieved from hubspot: http://blog.hubspot.com/marketing/psychology-of-stories-storytelling-formula#sm.0019nk9tb1634d2rzy114508pbvwf

Kuhlmann, S., Piel, M., & Wolf, O. (2005). Impaired memory retrieval after psychosocial stress in healthy young men. *Journal of Neuroscience, 25*(11), 2977–2982. doi:10.1523/JNEUROSCI.5139-04.2005.

Morris, W. (1969). *American heritage dictionary of the English langaue*. New York: American Heritage Publishing.

Pancner, K. (1978). The use of parables and fables in Adlerian psychotherapy. *Individual Psychologist, 15*(4), 19–29.

Schwabe, L., & Wolf, O. (2010). Learning under stress impairs memory formation. *Neurobiology of Learning and Memory, 93*(2), 183–188. doi:10.1016/j.nlm.2009.09.009.

Stocker, A. A., & Simoncelli, E. P. (2006). Noise characteristics and prior expectations in human visual speed perception. *Nature Neuroscience, 9*, 578–585.

Warnock, S. (1989). Rational-emotive therapy and the christian client. *Journal of Rational-Emotive & Cognitive-Behavior Therapy, 7*(4), 263–274.

Chapter 12
Treating Children with NCLT

NCLT is, in every sense, a model of the factors that contribute to the development of an individual's mental health. As such, it should go without saying that its principles apply to the development of these skills in children. With the addition of some caveats, the learning process of children is governed by the same principles as the learning process of adults. Therefore, NCLT treatment methodology can be, and is, routinely used with children and their families.

What are some of the caveats that therapists should be mindful of when working with children? The following is not meant to give an exhaustive view of a complex and extensive literature. It is intended to give the practitioner a starting point should they wish to explore this topic in detail.

Perspective Taking Is Different in Children

Children generally view the world more egocentrically than adults, and as a result, have more difficulty recognizing and accepting the perspectives of others (Epley, Morewedge, & Kaysar, 2004). This makes introducing the idea that others think differently more difficult and time consuming. Children develop perspective taking skills as they mature, because they are better able to subsequently correct an initial egocentric interpretation. This introduces a life course interpretation to the development of problems related to poor perspective taking in that it is not a matter of the development of problems, but rather it is a problem with the development or lack thereof of the skill of perspective taking. The NCLT model holds that problems related to failure in perspective taking are a matter of where people stop in the development of these skills, rather than deficiencies in where they start. The NCLT model posits that an ongoing egocentric bias among adults is produced by insufficient correction of an automatic moment of egocentrism that occurs naturally as part of a child's development.

© Springer International Publishing AG 2017 149
T. Wasserman, L.D. Wasserman, *Neurocognitive Learning Therapy: Theory and Practice*, DOI 10.1007/978-3-319-60849-5_12

Failure to perspective take, or poor ability to perspective take, has interesting mental health implications developmentally. Children who display more egocentricity tend to display more problems regulating executive function (Nilsen & Graham, 2009). Research suggests that children's inhibitory control skills allow them to inhibit their own perspective, enabling them to make use of their communicative partner's perspective. That is, children with effective inhibitory skills can regulate their perceptions better and be more open to the interpretation of others. Children with poor executive management skills tend therefore to be more egocentric and less open to the interpretation of others. These children go on to display more emotional and behavior regulation difficulties as they get older. In other words, these are the children you will see in your offices and this is why it is critical to teach perspective taking skills as part of treatment.

Executive Control Matures

Although the laws of learning that govern how people learn do not change, there are some critical differences between adults and children in how they learn. Basically, the process of learning comes to operate under increasing executive control in the years between middle childhood and early adulthood (Kuhn & Pease, 2006). Specifically, a major ability of executive management that develops in the years from childhood through adulthood is increasing meta-level monitoring and management of cognition (Kuhn, Katz, & Dean, 2004). This effectively implies that as we get older we are better able to decide what to focus on based upon factors other than novelty, threat, or immediate reward. We are more able to utilize distant reward considerations and include intangible reinforcers. That is, we are, if the process goes according to plan. For many of the people we see in our practices, this does not happen. The rewards they choose continue to be more immediate, and they tend to ignore rewards that are distant, or to come in the future. Children with ADHD are particulalrly susceptible to this type of pattern, and we have described how this difficulty in reward selection may contribute to the clinical picture typically encountered in ADHD (Wasserman & Wasserman, 2015).

Intuition and Its Power over Decision Making Develops over Time

Dual process theory provides a model that describes how a cognitive outcome can occur in two different ways, or more specifically, as a result of two different processes (Kahneman, 2011). Most dual processing theories describe these two processes as consisting of an implicit (automatic) process that is fast and efficient, and an explicit (cognitively controlled), conscious process. In line with NCLT modeling, explicit processes, especially highly verbalized ones, or attitudes and actions, can be changed through persuasion or education. Implicit process or attitudes, which are highly automated, usually take a long amount of time to change as they rely on the elimination of old habits and the formation of new habits that will become automated through intense training and practice. As might be expected, young children have fewer and less intensely developed implicit processes except for those that are biologically programmed. One of these processes is intuition, which is defined as processing without the benefit of purposeful cognitive input. Judgments/ decisions/choices that are eventually expressed are called intuitive if they retain the hypothesized initial automated proposal without much modification (Kahneman & Frederick, 2001). As a result of these routines building and becoming more complex over time, young children are less intuitive and more concrete. Children become more intuitive over time (Reyna, 2004). Acquired maladaptive attitudes and emotional response sets become more entrenched and automatic over time. Younger children are in this sense more cognitively flexible and more amenable for modification within the limitations of their level of cognitive development.

Working with Children Means Working with Their Families

The fact that we included the families in that statement points to the fact that when working with very young children the treatment emphasis changes a bit. It moves from intervention targeting entrenched maladaptive response sets to intervention designed to develop adaptive response sets that for one reason or another have not yet been automated. As with all types of learning, the acquisition of adaptive emotional response sets requires opportunities to learn, opportunities to practice, and opportunities to generalize. Adults can provide their own opportunities children, especially younger children need to have these opportunities provided for them. These opportunities are provided by parents and teachers. As a result both parents and teachers are intimately involved when young children are being treated. The idea that you can take a young child into an office and practice skills with them and not provide the opportunities for practice and generalization is contrary to the laws of learning and good NCLT practice.

For the NCLT practitioner, working with parents and teachers means that both the parents and teachers are trained to understand how children learn. In addition both parents and teachers use these skills in collaboration with the therapist and child to provide targeted learning opportunities designed to teach the skills. Here is a case example of how this is accomplished.

Mike

Mike is a 15–year-old young man with high functioning autism. He has been in treatment for some time and understands the NCLT model. He has been working on a variety of maladaptive responses. Most recently he has conquered difficulty in working with groups of students on projects that require cooperation. He has demonstrated a long history of having temper tantrums in groups when the other group members do not want to go along with his ideas. He believes his ideas are better and that they will all get better grades if they would but listen to him. This issue was resolved by putting in a strategy using a coping statement that had Mike think about and then make one statement to the group. If he could not persuade them, he would agree to follow the voted upon idea. To counter his anxiety regarding the grade and his worry that the teacher would not know that Mike knew the right way, Mike was permitted to write a short note to the teacher outlining his idea. The teacher agreed to receive the note and comment on it, and Mike agreed to accept the grade that the group earned on the project.

This series of issues clearly demarcated a central belief or response tendency that was a major problem for Mike. Mike is exceptionally intelligent. He frequently received scores in or above the 99th percentile on standardized tests and is capable of taking all of the accelerated classes that the school offers. His ability to do so is continually hampered by outbursts that he has in class. These outbursts are of such magnitude that Mike is accompanied by an aide to his classes so that intervention can be immediate if one of these outbursts were to occur. The outbursts all have a predictable trigger. Mike encounters a situation where he does not have an immediate answer available. This response set can occur in situations ranging from a direct question asked by the teacher to a question on an in seat assignment. If Mike does not know the answer, he will immediately ask to the teacher to explain it to him. If the teacher does not immediately respond to his question, Mike becomes agitated and disruptive. He becomes terrified that he does not know the answer because a good deal of his self-esteem is tied up in being the smartest kid in school. Mike believes that this status would be immediately removed if he did not know some piece of information.

In order to avoid these situations Mike has requested to be enrolled in the easiest classes in the grade as opposed to the harder AP classes. He believes that he will not be challenged in these classes but on the other hand he will get all of the questions right. Neither his parents nor his therapist believes that this is a judicious plan as it surely will mean that Mike will not gain entrance to the highly ranked university that he aspires to. Mike has agreed to try AP classes and just come to session after the first week of school to report that he has had another outburst in a classroom and was restrained by support staff. The AP teacher is indicated that, due to the pace of learning in the class, Mike's disruptions cannot be tolerated and he will have to drop down to easier classes if they continue.

By this time the central theme triggering Mike's responses has been identified, made clear, and articulated by Mike and his family; Mike believes that it is unacceptable to receive anything less than an A. When asked, he will explain that an A in a basic class is preferable to an A- in an AP class. He maintained this belief even after the local school districts scoring code is explained wherein the A- in an AP class would give him more points on his GPA than would an A in the basic class. While Mike is able to articulate that the AP class would help him more than the basic class, he maintains his preference for A's in the basic class.

Mike comes into session frustrated with himself. He states that he now recognizes that staying in the AP class is preferable, but he also understands that there will be things he does not know in the AP class. In fact, the recent outburst was triggered when the teacher looked over an assignment that Mike submitted and congratulated him on his work, but also suggested that additional analysis would yield a more sophisticated answer. Upon hearing this critique, Mike panicked and disrupted the class, forcing his removal.

Mike states that he is very aware of his response predisposition and that he frequently defaults to an anxiety response. He states that he cannot help himself. At this point there are a number of things that could have been attempted. Most of them would involve targeting the anxiety in response to the situation or perhaps cognitive disputation regarding the fact that not knowing was inherently threatening. These would be pragmatic solutions that might work, but in fact had not been successful. What was decided however was to teach a new response to "not knowing." Please remember that Mike had already been in NCLT-based treatment and understood that his maladaptive response represented a practiced choice to a trigger and that he would, if he desired and practiced, be able to train a new response. Mike was an active participant in his treatment and the problem solving it represented. He was the one who indicated that he needed a new "response schema" in these situations.

A discussion ensued, one which after a time his mother joined, in which the response of scientists to not knowing was reviewed. The idea of failed attempts was introduced, and a discussion followed that reviewed the number of failed attempts most scientists have on the way to their successes. Mike very much fashioned himself a scientist, and by redefining how scientists embraced unknowns, Mike was able to alter his schema. Then, together with the therapist and his parents, it was decided that the better response to unknowns would be excitement and inquisitiveness. Mike altered his schema and decided that in fact, he would never become a scientist if he did not adopt this view of the situation. Clearly, being a scientist was more important than other considerations. This discussion was followed by a contact with several of Mike's teachers by e mail wherein they assured Mike that he could still get A's even though he did not know everything before it was presented. Mike was not promised A's, he was only told that the opportunity still existed.

Mike agreed to try the new model. His parents agreed to offer opportunities for practice and reminders at home, and the teachers were contacted and agreed to offer reminders/prompts to Mike in class. These reminders were to take the form of "I am going to tell you something you may not know. Remember, this is an opportunity to be excited and inquisitive, and show me that you really want to learn new things." Opportunities were provided for mastery at home and in school. There were no extrinsic rewards utilized. Success and mastery was conceptualized as their own rewards. At the time of this writing Mike has gone several months without an outburst. There have been some close calls where he hesitated and struggled with applying his new response set. These new responses, however, are becoming increasingly automatic.

This example contains many of the elements that characterize NCLT process as regards children. Firstly, there is a clear emphasis on teaching and learning as well as a process to make implicit triggers explicit. I should point out that this is not the only way this case could have been handled. As we have pointed out, there could have been a focus on decreasing anxiety or managing anxiety by techniques such as relaxation. The important thing to recognize is that the client was an active participant in the process. From identifying the triggers to deciding from amongst options, the choices were largely his. This is because there was recognition by all the participants that unless he committed to the choices, real movement would not be made. It is also different than what would be expected in many therapy situations. Key individuals in Mike's life were very conversant with the target goals and were active participants in the treatment. The treatment and the work did not take place behind closed doors in isolation from the rest of the world. Treatment took place in the environment that required the new and adaptive behavior. This permitted in situ learning and generalization. Finally, to the developmental extent possible, the child understood what was being done and why. He learned about the things that were sustaining his maladaptive choices, and also learned about the model we were going to use to change them into adaptive choices and responses.

Parents and Teachers Are Effective Adjuncts for Therapy

There is a substantial body of research literature that indicates that parents and teachers are effective therapeutic agents for specific types of behavioral problems (McCart, Priester, Davies, & Azen, 2006). There is for example, research suggests that (1) therapy proved more effective for children than for adolescents, and (2) this was particularly true when the therapists were paraprofessionals (e.g., parents, teachers) or graduate students (Weisz, Weiss, Alicke, & Klotz, 1987) who were trained in a treatment model in order to provide their services. That is not to say that professionals were not successful, but it does say that trained paraprofessionals offered important support services for treatment. It is also important to note that NCLT is particularly didactic and suitable for this purpose. There are examples of training and orientation tools for both parents and teachers provided in the appendices of this volume. There are some additional findings from this research that should also be kept in mind. Specifically, individuals with professional degrees (doctor's or master's) were particularly effective in treating problems characterized by over controlling such as phobias or shyness, but were not more effective than other therapists in treating problems characterized by under regulation such as aggression or impulsivity. Finally, behavioral treatments proved more effective than nonbehavioral treatments regardless of client age, therapist experience, or treated problem. In short, therapists who ignore parents and teachers as effective teaching resources in therapy are failing to utilize an important resource.

NCLT is not the first therapeutic modality to consider the use of parents as collaterals in therapy. The Centers for Disease Control (CDC) advocates parents learning behavior management skills while their children undergo treatment with a professional for AD/HD (Centers for Disease Control and Prevention, 2016). These management skills, learned through a variety of programs, are to be used at home while the treatment regimen in the office remains separate. We do not argue with the idea that children, at times, need a safe place to discuss family issues and seek resolution. There are problems however that benefit from an integrated approach involving key persons in the child's life and at those times NCLT recognizes the benefit of having parents and teachers involved. In addition the generalizability of the training is enhanced when others in the child life are using the same principles and language to help shape behavior. NCLT practitioners purposefully integrate parent training into the therapeutic process. If done correctly and completely, this insures that the work will continue long after the contact with the professional has ended.

Building Resilience

As we have stressed NCLT is a model that describes a process in which a child develops a healthy emotional life. As such, it encourages the development of resilience. Resilience is defined as "the ability to adapt well to adversity, trauma, tragedy, threats or even significant sources of stress" (Alvord, Gurwitch, Martin, & Palomares, 2016). Resilient children tend to be emotionally healthy (Ginsberg, 2007) (Campbell-Sills & Stein, 2006). Being resilient means that children will be ready for times when they experience difficulty or distress. The American Psychological Association identifies that the following activities (Adapted from the Resilience Guide published by the American Psychological Association) encourage the development of resilience in children and these activates are included as part of NCLT therapeutic process.

1. **Children benefit from social connections**
   Children should be specifically taught skills that will help them make friends. Empathy should be one of the skills taught, including the skill of empathy, or feeling another's pain. Many of the children we see in treatment have difficulties in this area. They are isolated from their peers as a result of their behavior. If the child is in preschool, preschool teachers are an excellent resource in identifying classmates that would support a child in learning the necessary skills.
2. **Children learn by helping others:**
   Helping others is often the best way to acquire skills.

3. **Maintain a daily routine:**

   Children are creatures of routine. They thrive on predictability. Having a sense of control over one's routines develops resilience.

4. **Children need downtime:**

   Children as well as adults need to relax. Over focus on areas of difficulty negatively affects the development of competence in children. We frequently encounter parents whose children are having educational difficulties and whose days are completely filled with activities designed to remediate these difficulties. The child literally spends all day with activities that they find frustrating and somewhat demeaning. This negatively impacts resilience. Endlessly worrying or overfocusing on areas of weakness can be counterproductive. Make sure a child has time to have fun, and make sure that your child hasn't scheduled every moment of his or her life with no "downtime" to relax.

5. **Teach your child self-care:**

   Self-care increases competence and competence develops confidence. Competence and confidence supports the development of resilience.

6. **Set attainable goals:**

   Teach children to set reasonable and readily attainable therapeutic goals. Encourage small steps being taken every day so the child learns that they can planfully move towards their goals.

7. **Encourage the development of a positive self-view:**

   Routinely identify and have the child identify areas of success in handling difficult situations. This again stresses the competence that the child already possesses and supports the development of resilience.

8. **Teach the child to keep things in perspective:**

   Even when the child encounters emotionally difficult events, help the child look at the situation in a larger context. Young children will have difficulty in seeing beyond the present, but help them understand that the event will end. This will help them develop a sense of control.

9. **Help the child view circumstances as opportunity for growth:**

   Reinforce the child for coping during difficult times.

10. **Understand that change is going to happen:**

Change is universally understood as causing anxiety in many people. It is especially anxiety producing for children who often feel somewhat powerless over their lives. Understanding that it will happen provides a sense of predictability and control. Pointing out when change is expected to occur is an important aspect of treatment for children.

These are the things we are supposed to develop. How do things go awry?

Of Slot Machines and Brett: Answering the Question How Did My Child Get This Way?

Have you ever seen one of the old Las Vegas or Atlantic City style slot machines? They were called "one armed bandits" for reasons you can probably guess. One would put a coin in the coin slot, pull the arm, and the drums would rotate. When they stopped you found out if you lost, or won and how much. Needless to say, the number of times one won was very small compared to the number of times one lost. Yet, people sat at those machines all day gambling.

One armed bandits are a great way to understand the principle of variable reinforcement. Variable ratio reinforcement is a reinforcement pattern that provides reinforcement after an unpredictable number of responses that on average reinforce a certain percentage of the time. This schedule creates a steady, high rate of responding. If you *knew* that the machine was broken and would not pay out, you would not engage that machine. But, if it *may* pay out, or more importantly *has* paid out on occasion, one's gambling behavior actually increases. Often the betting increases in intensity because we are '*certain*' that the machine will reward us shortly. This is a wonderful metaphor for how we humans behave. Once we understand this learning principle, the possible corollaries are numerous. We are going to use it to demonstrate how maladaptive behaviors begin and are perpetuated in children.

Let's begin with Brett. Brett is 9 months old. Brett has been bottle fed, but his parent is now deciding it is time to wean him off the bottle. Brett, for the first time, gets put to bed without his bottle, and as we would predict, he now starts to cry. His parent ignores him. He cries louder. In a moment of empathy, his parent decides that Brett is not ready to give up his bottle and brings him his bottle. Brett is content and stops crying. However, the parent still believes that the bottle is no longer a good thing for Brett. They have made a mistake and want to try again. The next night they put Brett to bed without his bottle, but he cries again. Brett's parent gives him half a bottle so he won't cry. The next night Brett's parent is determined not to give Brett a bottle. Brett begins to cry, after all, that worked the previous nights. Brett's parent is determined and holds fast. What does Brett do now? Well, he doesn't stop crying. In fact, he cries harder and louder. As Brett's parent has to go to work in the morning and is just exhausted, they give him the bottle. The next night is easy to predict; Brett doesn't cry. Rather, Brett now screams, because crying louder and louder has paid off.

Unfortunately, we have now taught Brett two things. The first thing we have taught Brett is that engaging in what is undesirable behavior for us pays off. It got him his bottle. The second thing we have inadvertently taught Brett is how *not to handle* stress. That is, the course of normal child development involves encountering stressors. In fact, it is desirable to encounter stressors. Part of being able to become resilient involves learning how to accommodate to stress. For an infant or toddler this may involve learning to self soothe or accommodate. Some children do this very well. They suck on their fist or simply curl up and go to sleep. Brett was not provided with that experience. Brett was inadvertently taught to become highly, and negatively aroused without learning to self soothe. That is, Brett's neurophysiological system became highly aroused, and left there without Brett learning to reintegrate.

In fact, children demonstrate a constitutionally inborn ability to regulate stress and it varies from individual to individual. Some infants handle stress better than others (Compas, 1987). In addition, as the networks responsible for stress management develop in response to environmental interactions, they determine the efficiency of the individual to handle stress. In other words, as regulatory subsystems are integrated, general mechanisms of coping accumulate developmentally (Skinner & Zimmer-Gembeck, 2007). Furthermore, children who demonstrate inefficiency in coping with stress in infancy go on to demonstrate significantly higher rates of emotional problems as young adults (Eisenberg, Smith, & Spinrad, 2011).

Brett is now 4 years of age. He is with his parent in the supermarket. His parent is on line at the deli counter. Brett has spied a bag of candy and wants it. In case you did not already know, they always put the candy and attractive items where the kids can see and grab them. His ever dutiful parent says no, but Brett starts to scream. People are staring. His parent is mortified, and after holding out for a few minutes gives Brett the candy just so they can finish their shopping. Again, one problem is that we are reinforcing undesirable behaviors in Brett and most clinicians would focus on the (correct) notion that Brett's parent is (inadvertently) reinforcing tantrums. That would be correct. Brett would be getting reinforced for an inappropriate behavior. As an NCLT therapist you would be focusing on the interplay between the behavior Brett is being "reinforced" for and the effect on his connectome. What is he learning, how is he learning it, and what will it generalize to?

Brett is now 11. He is in the sixth grade. He likes his teacher. She is a good teacher. She is responsive to the children in her class. The teacher is in the middle of a lesson. Brett has a question. He raises his hand, but Miss Smith is ignoring him, so he blurts out the question. When Miss Smith attempts to quiet Brett, he yells his point. Miss Smith gives Brett an in class detention. Brett has to explain this to his parent and demonstrating his lack of repentance, insists to his parent that the teacher was not answering his question. He asserts "That is her job! She is supposed to answer my questions!" Although Brett's parent is aware of the correct social response, he/she is also somewhat torn. After all he's right, isn't he?

The answer of course is that he is *partly* right. A teacher is there to help answer questions. But Brett is asking the one armed bandit to pay off every time he pulls the lever. When it doesn't, he becomes very distressed and increases his behavior. In this case, the increased rate of responding is maladaptive. In NCLT terms, his coping mechanisms did not operate effectively, he had not learned to delay responding when the social situation required it, and he became over aroused and cannot reintegrate himself.

Brett is now 17. His parent is at their wits end and decides to bring Brett to therapy. Essentially, they want you to "fix him." At intake they explain that Brett has always been difficult, and lately verbally combative. When his parent attempts to correct him, he becomes even more argumentative. The parent explains that they have punished him by taking away everything they can think of. Except of course his car, because he is not registered for the school bus, that would take 2 weeks, and he has to get to school, and his phone because he may need it in an emergency. They explain that the typical problem scenario at home begins with Brett asking for something. The parent doesn't understand why Brett gets so upset when they have to sometimes say no. They think they are very generous with Brett and give him almost anything he wants. During these confrontations with Brett the parent will usually give up, defeated and angry. They describe Brett as selfish and nasty. If you work with teenagers you have seen some variant of this scenario. As an NCLT therapist you recognize that Brett is "playing the slots": Why not take a chance on getting away with increasingly problematic behaviors when the payout is use of a car and smartphone? It is however at this juncture more than just deciding to play. The overt cognitive decision was long ago eliminated and replaced with highly automated behavior that has developed as a result of these maladaptive responses being repeated, practiced, and often reinforced. Brett no longer has to think about this type of reactive behavior. It comes "naturally to him." Brett engages in the responses behaviorally and emotionally without cognitive effort of any sort. Some models might say that his personality is fully formed. We would just say that the learning cycle regarding the expression of this response pattern is complete.

The above scenario, or some part of it, is one we typically see in our clinical practices. Depending upon the age of the child, we usually help the parent implement behavior charts and reinforcement paradigms. That of course, is very important. As an NCLT therapist however, you recognize that this is important not only to improve behavioral compliance, but for two other reasons as well. Firstly, every clinician knows that implementing a behavior increases the likelihood of demonstrating that behavior again. An NCLT therapist understands that implementing *and practicing that behavior* improves its accessibility. It becomes a skill that we hope is practiced to the point of automaticity. The same way as when someone says "Good morning" to Brett, he responds in kind. He has practiced that interchange multiple times, to the point of automaticity. As an NCLT therapist you are selecting behaviors not only to secure compliance, but to make them automatic. Secondly, as an NCLT therapist, you recognize the impact of practicing positive, reinforcing behaviors on the emotional regulation networks. You are helping Brett to rework his connectome—to better be able to emotionally self-regulate.

In addition, as a good NCLT therapist you understand the interplay between appraisal and behavior. You understand that you need to explain to this parent how it is necessary to make it "rewarding" for Brett to engage in these behaviors. You also stress the importance of providing Brett with cognitive strategies and verbally based coping statements to help him better internalize and integrate these behaviors and values. They are all part of the network. You are working on the whole network.

A Word About Teenagers

Working with teenagers is of course a challenge. They are usually not the ones to choose to come for therapy and therapy can become just an extension of their rebelliousness. Perhaps they choose not to speak to you. After all, that was successful in getting rid of the last two therapists. We have found that by explaining our model, which is a learning one depathologizes the process for the teen ager and makes it more likely that they will agree to participate. We have also found that by telling the teenager that learning a new way of responding will get their parents "off their backs" is very persuasive in getting the teen to participate in the treatment. This is of course true, as teens improve in their responses to their parents, their parents frequently relax. Teens are often brought to therapy by exasperated parents who think that the teen is the problem. The teens understand this very well. Just in case anyone is confused about this, we will add that the teens do not agree. They view their parents as unreasonable, archaic and demanding. Sometimes this view might be independently evaluated as accurate. We try to enlist the teen to change the family pattern of behavior. While this inherently means that the teen will change some of their behavior, it also means that they will help you get the parent to change some of theirs. They are enlisted in an experiment. Some sign on because they think it will work and some sign on because they want to show you how intractable their parents can be. Nevertheless, most sign on. If this sounds a bit like a family system approach, that is because in this element it is. It is another way that NCLT is truly an integrative therapeutic approach.

As the NCLT therapists you will have multiple areas you can choose from in which to intercede. Perhaps one of the most important interventions in Brett's case was helping his parent to understand that Brett did not develop coping skills and as a result has no resilience. This is a very novel concept for a parent who is traditionally focused on their child's behavior rather than their neurophysiological integration. Imagine the difference in a parent trying to control their teenage child's behavior versus the parent trying to help their teenage child develop resilience. Perhaps as the NCLT therapist you decide to work with the parent to help them develop better *emotional* regulation in their child. Imagine the difference in the verbal exchanges—"You are ungrateful and nasty" vs "I know this is frustrating for you." Perhaps you decide to work with the teenage himself in order to help the teenager address his emotional dysregulation. Or help teach him a way to procure whatever he finds reinforcing by teaching him new behavioral and social skills. To recognize his schemas and triggers. Perhaps that is asking him why, if he hates this teacher so much, is he trying to spend more time with her next year by having to repeat the class after he fails it. Therapy then becomes about teaching Brett, and Brett learning how he can get what he wants (avoid another class with her). His solution just may involve how is he going to appraise the situation differently and perhaps chose the less arousing reinforcer (getting his work done) over a more arousing reinforcer (video games) and then reinforce himself for carrying out that plan?

In either event, we hope that this vignette has helped to demonstrate how behavior can be, sometimes inadvertently, shaped to become maladaptive response patterns. And how this behavior can result in not only behaviorally maladaptive patterns, but emotionally maladaptive patterns as well and finally how these learned patterns become the types of response patterns that are "diagnosed." We also hoped to highlight a major difference between NCLT and other models. In NCLT, emotion and behavior are not separable. They are the result of repeated expressions of the emotional and behavioral response patterns which become learned to the point of automaticity. They effect changes in the connectome. Our job is to restructure the connectome. Our job with parents and teachers is to have them no longer focus solely on the behavior, but rather on all of the aforementioned factors, have them state a goal, understand the implications of that goal, support and provide the skills to achieve it.

Being pediatric neuropsychologists and having worked with newborns and infants in neonatal intensive care has provided us with a unique perspective on the genesis of many behavioral and regulation difficulties. The case of Margret is a good example which we will use to illustrate the life course and learning emphasis found in NCLT.

Margaret

Mrs. Smith brings her daughter Margaret, who is 9 months of age, in to see you stating that she has come in because she is having difficulty getting her daughter to calm down at night and go to sleep. Mrs. Smith, who is clearly frazzled and somewhat sleep deprived, reports that Margaret would just cry and cry at night. She describes Margaret as a colicky and fussy baby. Mrs. Smith has consulted with her pediatrician who has diagnosed colic and recommended nonallergic formula as well as some additional steps. Margaret's parents tried allergy free formulas to no avail, however the act of nursing itself proved the most calming. Margaret's sleep difficulties persist, which has precipitated the visit to your office. Mrs. Smith is hoping to learn some behavioral techniques that would address Margaret's ongoing sleep difficulties. Mrs. Smith reports that Margaret calms when she is breast fed, but as soon as a parent tries to put down Margaret to sleep on her own, Margaret cries again. Her mom has to pick her up, cuddle her and for want of sleep, Margaret's mother lets her breastfeed again. Every time Mom successfully leaves the room, Margaret wakes up crying and Mom has to go back in anyway. After all, Dad has to get to work in the morning. He too needs his sleep. At this point, Margaret and her mother are essentially sleeping together. As long as Margaret can nurse, she is calm. The strain on the parent's relationship is escalating.

Margret is a good example of a child that can be considered from several perspectives. The perspective we accept is going to strongly influence how we determine who the client is in this instance, which for some of us would most likely end up being Margaret. Try to imagine what treatment approach you would take if

Margaret and her parents showed up in your office asking for help in getting Margaret to sleep. What additional questions might you have before you proceed? Specifically, what would your interventions be? As an NCLT therapist, how would you explain what is going on here and why you are choosing what you are choosing?

Additional questioning indicates that no, Margaret does not have any food allergies and yes, she is accepting food supplements. Her height and weight is well within normal limits. Interestingly, if Margaret's parents have to go out and Margaret's grandmother puts her to sleep, Margaret does fall asleep.

Aha! Instantly the first attribution is made and the first treatment target created. Clearly, this is a case of Margaret's mother reinforcing Margaret's nursing behavior. After all, why would Margaret fall asleep with her grandmother if this was not Margaret's mother's doing.

Perhaps as the therapist you now have other hypotheses. In the therapy world, explanations abound. Perhaps Margaret's mother does not wish to give up nursing. Perhaps she is inadvertently reinforcing Margaret's nursing behavior. Perhaps Margaret's mother does not want to sleep with Margaret's father and is using little Margaret as a shield literally and figuratively. Perhaps Margaret's mother, due to trauma of her own, is too afraid to let her daughter cry to not breastfeed. Clearly, you say, Margaret's mother is the key here. Be mindful of how your hypotheses affect your intervention strategies and, just as importantly, your beliefs about and attitude toward Margaret's mother.

After a good clinical interview you are satisfied that Margaret's mother is not avoiding her husband and really does want Margaret to sleep through the night. He does too. In fact, he keeps pointing out how his mother seems to not have any problem getting Margaret to sleep.

Certainly following each of the threads mentioned above goes beyond the capacity of this chapter to follow to its conclusion. What we again wish to highlight is the interplay of neurophysiology and environment that characterizes the NCLT perspective.

As a starting point, it is important to remember that children demonstrate a constitutionally inborn ability to regulate their emotional reactions to stress and that this ability to regulate and self soothe varies from individual to individual (Mangelsdorf, Shapiro, & Marzolf, 1995). As we noted previously, this implies that some infants handle stress better than others (Compas, 1987). There are also other characteristics of infants who demonstrate colic, are more easily frustrated, and are more difficult to soothe. Easily frustrated infants use different emotional regulation strategies and are considered less attentive and more active than less easily frustrated infants. These hard to soothe infants are also characterized by their parents as more active, less attentive, and more distressed to novelty. Infants classified as easily frustrated have been found to be more reactive physiologically and less able to regulate physiological reactivity than their less easily frustrated counterparts (Calkins, Dedmon, Gill, Lomax, & Johson, 2002). Taken together, these characteristics may in fact constitute a temperament type. Margaret may in fact be one of these children, and her reaction therefore, a typical one. One must always consider the possibility that these reactions were not caused solely based on the competence or incompetence of the parents.

Over time, the networks responsible for stress management in these individuals continue to develop in response to environmental interactions and that process determines the overall efficiency of the individual to handle stress. It is also important to remember that these environmental interactions are themselves shaped by the temperament of the individual experiencing them. As regulatory subsystems are integrated, general mechanisms of coping accumulate developmentally (Skinner & Zimmer-Gembeck, 2007). The results of this developmental, and perhaps epigenetic, interaction between the connectome and the environment can be quite far reaching. Children who demonstrate inefficiency in coping with stress in infancy demonstrate significantly higher rates of emotional problems as young adults (Eisenberg et al., 2011). As this information pertains to Margaret and her parents, this suggests that Margaret's interactions with her mother, father, and grandmother, combined with her inborn efficiency to self-regulate (soothe) is laying the groundwork for how efficiently Margaret is able to cope, or perhaps not cope, with stress later on in life. This will continue to impact her as she develops.

Given that there is a substantial heritability component for temperamental characteristics (Saudino, 2005), it is somewhat possible that Margaret's mother may have herself followed a similar progression in the acquisition of coping skills. As an NCLT therapist we must consider the possibility that Margaret's mother is less resilient, less efficient at handling stress.

Here again is a very powerful example of a difference in effect on a client; there is a very big difference between labeling, and calling a parent a bad parent, versus highlighting to them how their own ability to tolerate stress is affecting their ability to handle their daughter's stress. The interaction between parent and child is a reciprocal one, and not necessarily or even likely, to represent pathology. It represents the result of two individuals with poorly evolved coping skill development interacting with each other. Specifically, research has demonstrated that interactions between child and parent temperament dimensions predicted higher levels of externalizing, internalizing, and attention problems over and above the effects of these dimensions alone (Retter, Stanger, McKee, Doyle, & Hudziak, 2006).

We might also point out how the message from the father, that he needs sleep and that this problem does not occur when his mother takes care of Margaret, is adding to Margaret's mother's stress. She in turn becomes more agitated, feels more incompetent, and when Margaret becomes agitated, her mother is less efficient in soothing her, creating a cycle of increasingly poor resilience from both parent and child.

Treatment at this point would include educating the parents about difficult to soothe infants, as well as teaching the parents about a child's need for consistency, routine, and predictability. It would also include teaching the parent about how to foster resiliency in their child so that they would not feel as though they were not taking care of their child's needs. Of course you would work on improving little Margaret's ability to self-soothe (Volling, McElwain, Notaro, & Herrera, 2002). By doing these things you would be focusing them on the longer, developmental perspective. We often validate how a parent is feeling, and then offer a scenario that forces the parent to adjust their beliefs and attitudes somewhat. For Margaret's parents that might be imagining her as a 4-year old about to enter a preschool program. From a life course perspective we would pose the question as to how they wish for their child to be able to emotionally handle this new, and potentially anxiety producing experience.

For the purposes of our example, let us assume that Margaret's parents did not come for assistance at this time, but instead waited for things to percolate a bit.

Margaret is now 4 years old. Her parents are excited to enroll her in a half day preschool. This will allow Mom some freedom to do some things that are just too hard with Margaret around. When Margaret is around, Mom can barely leave the room! Margaret is fine when she is occupied, but as soon as she realizes that Mom is not around, she cries. It is very hard to get laundry done and beds made when you have to tote a 4-year old around. Margaret's mother is mostly ready for this milestone; however, she is a bit torn. This is a big step for both Margaret and for her mother. She and Margaret have not really been apart. But, Mom agrees that it is time for some separation. After all, her friends are doing the same with their children. Mom prepares Margaret. She tells her that she is going to a place to play with other children. Mom takes Margaret to the preschool, and like the other mothers, she sits in the back of the room so that the children can acclimate to the new setting while being able to see their parent. Margaret stays with her Mom. Her mom is somewhat embarrassed, and in an attempt to show that she really is a good mother, Margaret's mother gives her big hugs and brings over books and toys with which to engage Margaret. The next week is the time for parents to drop off their children, but not stay in the room. Margaret's mother tells her that Mommy is going to leave, but she will be back. She attempts to leave. Margaret is not happy. She cries. Mom comes back into the room and stays. They will try again tomorrow. Tomorrow comes and Mom again attempts to leave. She gives Margaret a very big, long hug and with tears in her eyes, assures Margaret that it will be OK. As it turns out, Margaret does not do well and the school suggests that perhaps she is not ready. Mom and Margaret go home to try again in kindergarten.

We are not suggesting that all 4-year olds need to be enrolled in a preschool program. We are suggesting that this is a portent of things to come. We are suggesting that a default emotional system is being developed that is maladaptive. We are suggesting that resilience is an ability to tolerate stress, and therefore a major necessary trait. Margaret has not, and is not being provided with opportunities to develop resilience. She has not developed the confidence to be on her own for short periods. She has not developed the assuredness that comes with predictability of a parent leaving and returning. She is not being provided with the opportunity to engage with others in a social setting, and to develop the skills that come with that exposure. She is having the groundwork for anxiety laid.

Margaret is now six. It is time for kindergarten. Margaret is not happy about this. Her mom assures her that it will be OK. She gives her long hugs to assure her. She also does her best to make certain that Margaret is safe. Mom talks to Margaret about stranger danger and safe touch many times. She wants to be certain that Margaret is safe. She brings her to school and Margaret sobs. One of the other children comes over to help soothe Margaret, and Margaret buries her face in her mother's lap and cries louder. The teacher approaches to help and Margaret swats at her, trying to get her to back away. Margaret's mother is shocked and embarrassed. Margaret has never done this before she assures the teacher. And in a way that is true; Margaret has had little opportunity to socially interact with peers and authoritative adults. She is terrified. After all, that is what she has been practicing, and that anxious response has become the highly automatic response.

An experienced therapist or teacher can assist Margret's mother in establishing a reward paradigm to get Margaret into class. The NCLT therapist is going to take the more comprehensive intervention approach. The NCLT therapist, in keeping in mind a child's developmental needs, is going to explain the concept of resilience to Margaret's mother so that Margaret's mother can understand what she is trying to build rather than get rid of (crying upon entering school). The NCLT therapist is going to help the teachers to build a successful paradigm wherein Margaret stays for brief periods of time, and gets to leave while she is still neurophysiologically integrated rather than when she has disintegrated and the mother needs to be called. The NCLT therapist is going to try to make certain that Margaret's mother is engaged in interventions at home with the same goal, helping Margaret to be on her own for short periods, successfully. For example, Margaret may be place in front of the TV to watch her favorite TV show and her mother will "suddenly remember" to check something in the car or kitchen. While this may be considered a neutral experience, it actually is the time for Margaret's mother to start building in coping statements and praise after the fact. That is, we know Margaret was distracted. We used it to maintain a low level of arousal. Under the condition of low arousal, Margaret successfully was able to stay on her own. Upon her return Margaret's mother will reinforce Margaret for her success (a process of backward chaining) thereby providing Margaret with a new database of successes to counteract the database of anxiety and disintegration. To Margaret's mother's delight, after a few weeks, when Margaret becomes anxious, her mother looks at her and reminds her that Margaret has handled this "hundreds" of times, offers multiple examples, and assures Margaret that this is just the same, she can handle this time too. Also to Margaret's mother's delight, after a few weeks Margaret is boasting to family and friends about her new friends at school.

Margaret is now 17. She is finishing high school soon and really wants to go on to college. The junior year at high school is very intense and anxiety producing. She's been really stressed. She wants to come to therapy to talk about this. Frankly, therapists may choose different styles to address her concerns. The NCLT therapist may also choose to focus on different aspects such as her emotions, her cognitions or peer and/or family pressures. The NCLT therapist will likely address all of these. The NCLT therapist will also depathologize her stress reactions, explain how they developed, how they are being maintained through her constitution, her experiences and her connectome, and then help her to manage it all. The NCLT therapist will address helping Margaret to keep things in perspective, help in understanding that change is going to happen and help Margaret view these experiences as opportunities for growth.

References

Alvord, M., Gurwitch, R., Martin, J., & Palomares, R. (2016). *Resilence guide*. Retrieved from American Psychological Association: http://www.apa.org/helpcenter/resilience.aspx

Calkins, S., Dedmon, S., Gill, K., Lomax, L., & Johson, L. (2002). Frustration in infancy: Implications for emotion regulation, physiological processes, and temperament. *Infancy, 3*(2), 175–197.

Campbell-Sills, L. C., & Stein, M. (2006). Relationship of resilience to personality, coping, and psychiatric symptoms in young adults. *Behaviour Research and Therapy, 44*(4), 585–599. doi:10.1016/j.brat.2005.05.001.

Centers for Disease Control and Prevention. (2016, August 11). *Attention dreficit/hyperactivity disorder*. Retrieved from Centers for Disease Control and Prevention: http://www.cdc.gov/ncbddd/adhd/treatment.html

Compas, B. (1987). Coping with stress during childhood and adolescence. *Psychological Bulletin, 101*(3), 393–403. doi:10.1037/0033-2909.101.3.393.

Eisenberg, N., Smith, C., & Spinrad, T. (2011). Effortful control: Relations with emotional regulation, adjustment and socialization in childhood. In K. Vohs & R. Baumeister (Eds.), *Handbook of self-regulation: Research, theory, and applications* (2nd ed., pp. 263–283). New York: Guilford Press.

Epley, N., Morewedge, C., & Kaysar, B. (2004). Perspective taking in children and adults: Equivalent egocentrism but differential correction. *Journal of Experimental Social Psychology, 40*(6), 760–768. doi:10.1016/j.jesp.2004.02.002.

Ginsberg, K. (2007). The importance of play in promoting healthy child development and maintaining strong parent-child bonds. *Pediatrics, 119*(1). doi:10.1542/peds.2006-2697. Retrieved from http://pediatrics.aappublications.org/content/119/1/182.full.

Kahneman, D. (2011). *Thinking, fast and slow* (1st ed.). New York: Farrar, Straus and Giroux.

Kahneman, D., & Frederick, S. (2001). *Representativeness revisited: Attribute substitution in intuitive judgment*. Retrieved from Research Gate: https://www.researchgate.net/profile/Shane_Frederick/publication/229071271_Representativeness_revisited_Attribute_substitution_in_intuitive_judgment/links/54087a8c0cf2c48563bd6c75.pdf

Kuhn, D., Katz, J., & Dean, D., Jr. (2004). Developing reason. *Thinking & Reasoning, 10*(2), 197–219. doi:10.1080/13546780442000015.

Kuhn, D., & Pease, M. (2006). Do children and adults learn differently. *Journal of Cognition and Development, 7*(3), 279–293. doi:10.1207/s15327647jcd0703_1.

Mangelsdorf, S., Shapiro, J., & Marzolf, D. (1995). Developmental and temperamental differences in emotion regulation in infancy. *Child Development, 66*(6), 1817–1828. doi:10.1111/j.1467-8624.1995.tb00967.x.

McCart, M. R., Priester, P. E., Davies, W. H., & Azen, R. (2006). Differential effectiveness of behavioral parent-training and cognitive-behavioral therapy for antisocial youth: A meta-analysis. *Journal of Abnormal Child Psychology, 34*, 527–543. doi:10.1007/s10802-006-9031-1.

Nilsen, E., & Graham, S. (2009). The relations between children's communicative perspective-taking and executive functioning. *Cognitive Psychology, 58*(2), 220–249. doi:10.1016/j.cogpsych.2008.07.002.

Retter, D., Stanger, C., McKee, L., Doyle, A., & Hudziak, J. (2006). Interactions between child and parent temperament and child behavior problems. *Comprehensive Psychiatry, 47*(5), 412–420. doi:10.1016/j.comppsych.2005.12.008.

Reyna, V. (2004). How people make decisions that involve risk. *Current Directions in Psychological Science, 13*(2), 60–66. doi:10.1111/j.0963-7214.2004.00275.x.

Saudino, K. (2005). Behavioral genetics and child temperament. *Journal of Developmental and Behavioral Pediatrics, 26*(3), 214–223.

Skinner, E., & Zimmer-Gembeck, M. (2007). The development of coping. *The Annual Review of Psychology, 58*, 119–144. doi:10.1146/annurev.psych.58.110405.085705.

Volling, B., McElwain, N., Notaro, P., & Herrera, C. (2002). Parents' emotional availability and infant emotional competence: Predictors of parent-infant attachment and emerging self-regulation. *Journal of Family Psychology, 16*(4), 447–465. doi:10.1037/0893-3200.16.4.447.

Wasserman, T., & Wasserman, L. (2015). The misnomer of attention deficit hyperactivity disorder. *Applied Neuropsychology: Child, 4*(2), 116–122. doi:10.1080/21622965.2015.1005487.

Weisz, J., Weiss, B., Alicke, M., & Klotz, M. L. (1987). Effectiveness of psychotherapy with children and adolescents: A meta-analysis for clinicians. *Journal of Consulting and Clinical Psychology, 55*(4), 542–549. doi:10.1037/0022-006X.55.4.542.

Chapter 13
Future Directions

Like many new models, NCLT faces the challenge of empirical validation both of the model of the development of mental health and the related clinical intervention system. To accomplish this it will be necessary to conduct research into the model of mental health that is the basis of NCLT. As we have outlined in this volume and elsewhere (Wasserman & Wasserman, 2016) the components of the model have been amply researched and validated. The unique combination that represents NCLT has not. The literature on the Life Course model will be instructive in this regard as that model outlines on a macro or systems level what NCLT talks about on a neurophysiological level. The models are symbiotic in that regard. There is emerging literature to substantiate the NCLT position that learning alters white matter (Scholz, Klein, Behrens, & Johansen-Berg, 2009) and neural architecture (Zatorre, Fields, & Johansen-Berg, 2012). White matter (myelin) has been demonstrated as an etiological factor in a wide range of psychiatric disorders, including depression and schizophrenia. "We now know that myelination continues for decades in the human brain; it is modifiable by experience, and it affects information processing by regulating the velocity and synchrony of impulse conduction between distant cortical regions. Cell-culture studies have identified molecular mechanisms regulating myelination by electrical activity, and myelin also limits the critical period for learning through inhibitory proteins that suppress axon sprouting and synaptogenesis" (Fields, 2008) (p. 361). These findings represent a solid foundation, and future research will have to demonstrate specific patterns of connectivity that are related to known issues with mental health. It is highly unlikely that just one pattern of connectivity will be related to such complex issues such as depression, so it will be just as important to identify the key network connectivity problems that are reflective of the patterns of learning that produce disorders of mental health. We need to be open to the fact that there may be no "smoking gun," no one or group of patterns that reflect a mental illness but rather, as life course theory, suggests a pattern of learned interactions that produce a maladaptive outcome. If that is the case, there will be as many patterns of network connectivity as there will be patterns of learned experiences leading to a specific outcome.

© Springer International Publishing AG 2017   169
T. Wasserman, L.D. Wasserman, *Neurocognitive Learning Therapy: Theory and Practice*, DOI 10.1007/978-3-319-60849-5_13

Flexibility Is Problematic as Regards Empirical Validation

An additional area of question to be answered actually lies in an area of NCLT strength, namely is its flexibility. But how does one empirically verify a model encompassing so many interchangeable variables. The answer is that the model is based on neuroscience and the neuroscience will validate both the premise of NCLT and its application consisting of various techniques. As the model is verified, its theoretical application permits a very flexible approach to the process of ameliorating specific sets of maladaptive behaviors. Differing combinations of therapeutic interventions may be utilized to achieve the same ends depending on the nature of the trigger and the processing style of the client. This should not be unexpected as, if you follow a life course model for the development of mental health, it becomes easy to conjecture a large number of environmental exigencies that would contribute to similar therapeutically defined outcomes. NCLT does recognize that validation becomes problematic, however, when you attempt to empirically validate a treatment approach based on the conception that specific interventions composed of specific elements must be used to treat a disorder in order to do the appropriate comparisons necessary to establish efficacy. The difficulty inherent in NCLT validation is not only the flexibility of its applications, it is that NCLT crosses disciplines.

Carter (2008) identified a number of problems inhernet in flexible approaches. He discussed the use of flexible batteries of neuropsychological tests in clinical setting.

In a clinical setting, a flexible battery of neuropsychological tests is very analogous to flexible treatment approaches in the problems their use creates for empirical validation. A flexible neuropsychological battery involves the use of a large variety of tests used in varying combinations. While each test is standardized, the battery is not. The exact group of tests chosen is dependent on the neuropsychologist's perception of the patient's presenting complaints. Although there are many similarities, there is no one flexible battery shared by all neuropsychologists. The same neuropsychologist may use different combinations of tests with different patients, or even a different combination of tests with the same patient at different assessments when repeated assessments are performed. As would be the case for clinician selecting specific treatment approaches for each trigger, neuropsychologists using this approach are creating their own unique test batteries with each administration, and are hoping that the fact that each of the individual tests, which are valid to some degree, will somehow validate the use of the entire battery. Most neuropsychologists understand that this logic is an error, and in essence, you can never empirically validate the entire battery albeit each component is valid to talk about the specific thing that it measures. The exact set of issue exists when a flexible clinical approach is utilized. Carter identified the following set of specific problems:

Problems with a Flexible Battery in Forensic Context

1. Different procedures for nearly every patient.
2. Different procedures across different examiners.
3. Nearly impossible to scientifically validate for sensitivity and specificity.
4. Extremely limited scientific evidence for its use.
5. Open to examiner bias in method selection rather than demonstrated accuracy.
6. Selection is made based on subjective complaints.
7. The value of the procedure on the validity of the patient complaints.

Carter concludes his review by noting that there is scant data available to guide the clinician's choice when assembling a flexible battery. Personal preference, economic factors, availability of specific training in the clinic, and other unscientific sources of examiner bias may dictate selection.

In the end, the fixed versus flexible argument is tied to the same issues as is the eclectic argument for clinical psychological treatment. To opt for a single treatment method composed of fixed and immutable components implies that the approach would address all of the issues that pertain to the development of an individual's mental health. For example, if one postulates that thoughts cause feelings then a system that is designed to change thoughts should work all the time. On a macro level that might be true, but a closer look at network connectivity indicates that specific thoughts are related to specific feelings dependent upon the history of the individual. Therefore, just changing a thought might not change an automatic feeling state produced by multiple exposure and practice. To do that you need to understand the trigger for the behavioral response and practice the adaptive solution. You need to do that because that will enable you to use the same techniques the next time you meet a similar situation. It is true that, on a functional level, cognitive behavior therapists have understood this for a long time. NCLT believes that understanding the underlying neuropsychological processes that explain why this happens will lead to more effective treatment. Only time and further research will tell.

References

Carter, S. (2008). *Neuropsychological assessment: Flexible or fixed? Discover your best option for the most valid results.* Retrieved from Claims Management; Strategies for Successful Resolution: http://claims-management.theclm.org/home/article/neuropsychological-assessment-flexible-or-fixed

Fields, R. (2008). White matter in learning, cognition and psychiatric disorders. *Trends in Neuroscience, 31*(7), 361–370. doi:10.1016/j.tins.2008.04.001.

Scholz, J., Klein, M., Behrens, T., & Johansen-Berg, H. (2009). Training induces changes in white-matter architecture. *Nature Neuroscience, 12*, 1370–1371. doi:10.1038/nn.2412.

Wasserman, T., & Wasserman, L. (2016). *Depathologizing psychopathology.* New York: Springer.

Zatorre, R., Fields, R., & Johansen-Berg, H. (2012). Plasticity in gray and white: Neuroimaging changes in brain structure during learning. *Nature Neuroscience Review, 15*, 528–536. doi:10.1038/nn.3045.

Chapter 14
Endnote: How We Got Here

What is NCLT? What is it that makes it important? What makes it unique? And lastly, how do I practice NCLT? These are the questions which we are trying to answer with the current publication. We believe that it is the means to making therapy relevant and empirically valid. It is a foundational marriage between neuroscience and clinical therapy. And it focuses on mental health rather than mental illness. It deconstructs diagnoses and reframes what the therapeutic focus should be, respecting and integrating from a life span perspective, what a person brings to therapy in terms of their neurophysiology and behavioral history.

NCLT was the therapeutic outcome of a lifetime journey for two psychologists who had the benefit of each other to serve as sounding boards, to help process cases and research studies, and to motivate each other to keep trying to make both ourselves and our field better.

Both Drs. Wasserman started out as purely pediatric psychologists. That was somewhat of an unconventional journey as at that time. Pediatric Psychology was first described as a research specialty in the late 1960s (Mesibov, 1984). One of the earliest examples Mesibov cites is the work of Don Routh (1982) focusing on hyperactivity. Jerome Kagan (1965) is credited with having specifically articulated the role a psychologist might play. He defined an interface between pediatric facets and psychology such as the early detection of childhood disorders and the application of theoretical and empirical knowledge to therapeutic intervention. The future of pediatric psychology became the application of research onto intervention (Mesibov, 1984).

Pediatric psychologists often worked in interdisciplinary settings along with psychiatrists and pediatricians. That applied to us, but with a significant enhancement; In addition to our private practices setting in an upper class area, we ran a Day Treatment Center in the City of New York for children who had been expelled from special education, or were being released from inpatient units. These children were from low SES backgrounds and often were exposed to the traumas associated with low SES, single parenting homes, etc. These children ranged in age from three to 18. Our job was to provide psychological services, employ applied psychology

© Springer International Publishing AG 2017   173
T. Wasserman, L.D. Wasserman, *Neurocognitive Learning Therapy: Theory and Practice*, DOI 10.1007/978-3-319-60849-5_14

techniques, and help these children successfully navigate an educational environment while at the same time learning to successfully and adaptively cope with environments that were often quite traumatic. The diagnoses ranged from conduct disorder, to Williams Syndrome, to schizophrenia.

Because of the age range, we needed to know about developmental psychology across a large part of a child's life span. Because of the inclusion of genetic disorders with this population we needed to consider child development, the recognition of and impact of genetic disorders, and the interplay of a child's individual constitution in conjunction with their environment. We quickly learned to give strong consideration to the backgrounds including socio-economic factors, parenting issues, learned patterns the children and teenagers came to us with, and those they continued to practice. We understood that we were competing with all of these factors as we tried to replace their maladaptive effects. We learned the value of reinforcement and motivation on a person's behavior and to recognize that these were often idiosyncratic. For example, we knew we could not compete using a token reinforcer system in terms of monetary value – some of these kids were selling stolen brass pipes from abandoned buildings for far more than we could ever reinforce them with some token items. In fact, they often made more than we did given the week.

What we came to learn is that these kids had a mind set (schema) from which they were operating: Life was unpredictable and punishing, so you had to take what you could get it when you could get it. So we changed their schema. We gave them predictability and safety. We always provided a chance for restitution when they had a problem, whether it was clashing with staff or not being able to finish their homework because the police were at their house most of the night. They had to resolve their issue with the staff and they had to sit down and do their homework. The result, almost every one of those kids came to the Day Treatment Center almost every day. We believe it was because it gave them a valued new schema wherein they had some predictability and security, and adaptive ways to handle adversity when it presented. And isn't that the essence of mental health.

The work was rewarding and it was exhausting. Deciding it was time for a personal change, we relocated, and moved into the world of Early Intervention, working with children between birth and 3 years of age. We improved our ability to help identify presentations of medical and genetic symptoms to our toolkits. We became Brazelton assessment trained (Als, Tronick, Lester, & Brazelton, 1977), learning how to recognize what a neonate was telling us about their resilience, ability to reintegrate and tolerate stress. We learned to look for clues such as a child's ability to tolerate noise, light, or touch, whether remaining neurophysiologically integrated, or decompensating and averting. We learned to look for sensory and motor coordination. We now better covered the spectrum from birth through young adulthood.

When we evaluated children for the schools, we came to realize that educators had little time nor use for many of the diagnoses and recommendations we, as a field, were providing. In fact, the diagnosis often became the label explaining away many of the symptoms psychologists and educators need to be addressing, thereby underserving the child. Parents across the nation began to withhold evaluations from the schools in order to avoid the labeling and subsequent trajectories. We understood that the value of an evaluation had to include more than metrics, and more than a label. We understood that it had to provide meaningful information about how that child processes information and functions. In short, we understood that we had to look at a child's neurophysiology and its impact on their functioning, and their learned patterns of behavior and its impact on their functioning. Each child, while possibly sharing a diagnosis, came with their own unique and idiosyncratic schemas. We learned that just providing a number quantifying how far behind a child was in the acquisition of reading skills was no substitute for telling a school why that child was not acquiring those skills in the first place. We studied the development of reading and mathematics skills and learned how to assess these skills from the standpoint of functionality. Helping the children, their parents, and their educators understand what was going on and *why*, was therapeutic.

Working with adults showed us how the aforementioned factors, early childhood, stressors, genetics, neurophysiogical integrity, and behavioral patterns became fashioned into automated routines that resulted in people playing out schemas over and over again, some of which were adaptive, and some of which were not. We came to understand that the reason we were having trouble selecting a diagnosis code was because we were not treating a child's refusal to do homework, or a faulty cognition, or a marital relationship problem. We were addressing the schemas people had developed to adapt to their environments and were repeating over and over, across settings, cognitions, feelings, and time. We came to understand the interplay of all of the aforementioned factors on neural processing in the brain, and how changes to the brain continue the maladaptive patterns or emotional sequelae. Remaining true to our roots, we relied more and more on understanding the interplay of life span development, a person's personal constitution and the cause and effect of neurophysiology. We understood that labeling a behavior or diagnosis was insufficient. We began to explain what we knew to our patients. We began to teach our patients how they learned those behaviors that were troubling them and we began to show them how to acquire new and adaptive behaviors while at the same time ridding themselves of the maladaptive routines that had brought them to treatment. We spoke about learning, not pathology, and our patients got better. Not only did they get better, they knew why they got better and were able to take that learning with them to new life situations.

We believe that we need to educate our clients, directly, through their families or through their educators, as to what we have learned so that they can apply it to their lives and situations. We call this process neurocognitive learning therapy—NCLT. We recognize that it is different, and that in order to be able to do it some strongly held convictions have to be put aside. Not the least of these is that every maladaptive action on the part of a person does not represent pathology. Maladaptive responses are an integral part of learning. It is only when they become the default automated responses that they become problematic.

About 10 years ago we began to appreciate the implications of integrated brain network models for our work. Understanding how the brain processed information led us to examine how that brain was processing information in therapy and for children, in school. We began to understand that the compartmentalized models of diagnosis no longer adequately represented what was transpiring with our clients. We began applying what we knew about neuropsychology and neurophysiology to how we worked with our clients. At first we did this within the context of the cognitive behavioral models we were trained in, but we began to understand that we could extend beyond those models and develop a model for the development of mental health. If we could understand how things were supposed to work, it would help us understand what was happening when things went awry. The result of that work was our first book *Depathologizing Psychopathology* (Wasserman & Wasserman, 2016), where we laid out our model. We hope we have demonstrated in this volume how to take that theory, and put it into practice. We hope you will try NCLT, and learn first-hand how powerful and effective the treatment is.

References

Als, H., Tronick, E., Lester, B., & Brazelton, T. (1977). The Brazelton neonatal behavioral assessment scale (BNBAS). *Journal of Abnormal Child Psychology, 5*(3), 215–229.

Kagan, J. (1965). The new marriage: Pediatrics and psychology. *American Journal of Diseases of Childhood, 110*, 272–278.

Mesibov, G. B. (1984). Evolution of pediatric psychology: Historical roots to future trends. *Journal of Pediatric Psychology, 2*, 15–17.

Routh, D. K. (1982). Pediatric psychology as an area of scientific research. In I. Tunia (Ed.), *Handbook for thepraclice of pediatric psvchology* (pp. 290–320). New York: Wiley.

Wasserman, T., & Wasserman, L. (2016). *Depathologizing psychopathology*. New York: Springer.

Appendices: Practice Handouts and Forms

The forms and handouts in this appendix are provided for you to use in your practice. They are designed to enhance the use of neurocognitive learning therapy by communicating with your patients, their families and schools about the nature of the treatment they are receiving and the role these important collateral people play in the ongoing treatment of your client.

We have found that educating important collaterals about how neurocognitive learning therapy works allows everyone in the environment to collaborate in producing an appropriate outcome. In our experience, teachers and parents often wish to know what is happening in the course of treatment. These handouts are designed to provide them with the information they need to have in order for them to be a contributing member of the treatment team for their child.

Appendix A: Teacher Orientation to Neurocognitive Learning Therapy

What Is Neurocognitive Learning Therapy?

Neurocognitive learning therapy (NCLT) is a therapeutic system designed to work with, and make use of, our understanding of how the human brain possesses and learns information. NCLT recognizes the importance of a child's experiences in the classroom and attempts to form an alliance of people important to any child, and have that alliance address issues in a consistent, reasonable, and scientifically based manner. NCLT is a developmental and holistic approach to intervention, recognizing that each person is a result of genetics, history, background, memories, etc. NCLT then represents a fusion of information processing theory, brain network models, and cognitive behavioral treatment models. It also permits the incorporation of other therapeutic techniques in a task-dependent fashion. Working with

© Springer International Publishing AG 2017
T. Wasserman, L.D. Wasserman, *Neurocognitive Learning Therapy: Theory and Practice*, DOI 10.1007/978-3-319-60849-5

teachers allows a child to receive the healthy messages, and practice the healthy behaviors we are trying to get them to learn, across people and across settings, in very much the same way we teach children of different ages and abilities, and help them to master the material.

What Is the Neurophysiological Basis of NCLT?

As an educational professional you understand that the learning processes used in the classroom are the same processes that your students use to learn in the world. While there may be unique subject matter to be learned in therapy, the processes you use to learn that subject are identical to those in use in the classroom. A basic premise of NCLT is that all learning occurs the same way. Whatever the subject, issue or person and emotional valence thereof, learning occurs over the same neural networks and is subject to the same laws governing working attention, processing efficiency, memory allocation, expression, and engagement. All environmental experiences provide the opportunity to learn (automatize) adaptive behavior. This is obviously not a surprise to an educational professional.

Understanding this makes it possible to develop a set of principles that would facilitate learning within the therapeutic environment that can translate into the classroom as well. These principles of learning will be quite familiar to you. The experiences we provide in therapy to facilitate learning are designed to provide the opportunity to unlearn (deautomatize) maladaptive behavioral or emotional responses to various environmental exigencies, and to learn, or relearn, more adaptive behaviors and emotional responses. How this expedited learning occurs in an environment where an individual is seeking to address issues related to mental health (therapy) is at the core of NCLT.

NCLT Is a Unique System

NCLT is not a type of therapy. It is a system of therapy. The therapeutic principles that form the core of NCLT actually underlie the functionality of every other therapeutic modality. As such, it represents the common core of all therapeutic techniques. This permits and supports the use of many other therapeutic techniques within NCLT practice. The goal of NCLT is to appropriately target the area of needed intervention. Sometimes this will be behavioral. Sometimes this will address emotion. Sometimes it means understanding a child from a genetic or life event perspective.

NCLT is as much an educational experience as it is a therapeutic model. The concepts and skills that are central to NCLT are taught to individuals.

Table A.1 Disorders whose symptomology are alleviated by memory reconsolidation

Attention deficit/hyperactivity disorder	Anxiety	Anger
Attachment disorder	Compulsive behavior	Depression
Guilt	Low arousal	Low motivation
Low self-worth	Poor motivation	Posttraumatic stress disorder
Perfectionism	Panic attacks	Phobic responses

The Basics of NCLT

1. The Principle of Memory Reconciliation

Prevailing wisdom was that learning that occurred in the presence of strong emotion became locked permanently into subcortical implicit memory circuits by special synapses never to be unlocked. It was permanently wired and would always be evoked when something happened. This meant that people had to accept that they could never change the way that they react to things, and that they just had to get used to it and adjust accordingly.

Recently, three independent groups of researchers converged on the conclusion that a wide variety of different psychotherapies can be integrated via their common ability to trigger the neurobiological mechanism of memory reconsolidation in such a way as to lead to deconsolidation of a previously learned emotional response. This is an important finding because it was amongst the first research findings that therapy can actually change the way we emotionally react to specific environmental events.

Instead, for the first time, researchers, using a specific therapeutic technique, one incorporated into NCLT, had been able to activate a learned emotional response and under certain conditions, found that its previously locked neural circuit had temporarily shifted back into an unlocked, de-consolidated, labile, destabilized, or plastic state. This unlocked state allowed prior maladaptive learning to be completely nullified, along with behavioral responses it had been driving. The temporarily labile circuit soon consolidates once again, returning to a locked condition. The researchers named this newly discovered type of neuroplasticity memory reconsolidation.

Research has identified a number of clinical conditions whose symptomology is alleviated by memory reconsolidation that occurs as part of NCLT (Table A.1).

Based on this research it is clear that the consolidation of emotional memory is not a one-time, finite process resulting in indelible emotional learning. This new knowledge forms the neuropsychological and neurophysiological basis for neurocognitive learning therapy. Clinically, this means that counteracting and regulating unwanted acquired responses are not the way to resolve emotional issues. Rather, relearning the adaptive response is.

NCLT is designed to teach adaptive emotional responses using well-established principles of learning, working in conjunction with specific empirically valid therapeutic techniques. As such it represents a truly integrated approach that is based on known science as regards neuropsychology, neuroplasticity, neurophysiology, and learning.

Requirements for De-consolidation: Reactivation Plus Mismatch

In order for the memories associated with emotional respondency to be de-consolidated, critical experience must take place when the emotional memory and related behavioral response is first reactivated. This critical experience should consist of perceptions that sharply mismatch or deviate substantially from what the reactivated target memory expects and predicts about how the world functions. This is what happens in therapy. Clinically, the mismatch can be either a full contradiction or disconfirmation of the target memory or a novel, salient variation relative to the target memory. If the target memory is reactivated by familiar cues but not concurrently mismatched, synapses do not unlock and reconsolidation is not induced. The classroom is a perfect environment for introducing perceptions that sharply mismatch the memory and associations interfering with the child's mental and academic health.

A three-step process is initially required in order to carry out the sequence eliminating the maladaptive memory and program a new adaptive memory and related behavior.

1. Symptom identification. Actively clarify with the client, or child, what to regard as the presenting symptom(s). These include the specific behaviors, somatics, emotions, and/or thoughts that the client wants to eliminate and when they happen.
2. Retrieval of target learning into explicit awareness, as a visceral emotional experience, the details of the emotional learning or schema underlying and driving the presenting symptom.
3. Identification of disconfirming knowledge. Identify a vivid experience (past or present) that can serve as living knowledge that is fundamentally incompatible with the model of reality in the target emotional learning retrieved in step 2, such that both cannot possibly be true. The disconfirming material may or may not be appealing to the client as being more "positive" or preferred. What matters is that it be mutually exclusive with the target learning. It may be already part of the client's personal knowledge, or may be created by a new experience.

There is a fourth step wherein the client verifies the new emotional response by generalizing it into new situations and contexts.

2. Reward Recognition

Estimates vary, but it has been suggested that human adults make 35,000 remotely conscious decisions each day. Assuming 16 waking hours each day that's almost 2200 decisions every hour, 36 decisions every minute, and 1 decision about every second and a half. Young children make as few as 3000 decisions in a day. Decisions represent choices between two or more options. That's what your student is doing when they choose between doing their homework and playing their favorite video game. They are making a choice between two options. These decisions are not isolated instances. Each one builds upon the other. These compounded choices not only build upon each other, they act interdependently with other contextually relevant decisions resulting in a complex web of interconnected patterns of actions and emotional responses.

Some decisions are practiced so much that they become automatic; we do them without having to think about them. After some practice we no longer think about them individually, they automatically occur in a sequence.

NCLT teaches that when a person is confronted by making a choice between two or more stimuli, a separate sampling process for each attribute of each of the available choices is conducted. When we are thinking about deciding between choices, our attention switches from one attribute consideration to the next. The order in which attributes are considered, as well for how long each attribute is considered (attention time), influences the predicted choice probabilities and choice response times. Both order of attribute consideration and attention time given to each attribute are important targets for discussion within an NCLT session.

Perceived rewards are a critical part of the consideration of choice attributes. For NCLT, understanding the value of rewarding and punishing stimuli from your child's perspective will enable an understanding of when and where such rewards and punishments will be identified and used. Helping your student identify potentially rewarding aspects of the desirable choice you wish them to make is an important part of the work in NCLT.

The Role of the Educator

Educators can be valuable in this process because they can help identify many of the targets to practice as well as many of the disconfirming events. They can identify maladaptive responses (emotional or behavioral) that are causing the individual student difficulty. Then, working in conjunction with the NCLT therapist, they can help by recognizing situations in the classroom that call for the adaptive response and cuing the student to engage in it. Teaching professionals can also point out the inconsistencies between the student's original perception and the realities in the classroom. Many times in therapy, situations that produce maladaptive responses can only be discussed because the situations arise in the student's everyday life outside of the therapy environment. Teachers are uniquely qualified to both identify these events and support the elimination of maladaptive responses and the relearning of adaptive ones by cuing those adaptive responses to occur. An NCLT therapist will actively work with professional educational staff to both obtain the targets for modification and plan for a teacher response that will facilitate new learning.

What Happens in Therapy?

NCLT Is About Learning

From an NCLT perspective a therapist assumes an active, instructive, and authoritative role and teaches patients to think and conduct themselves differently. This is initially a collaboration between the therapist and the client with the therapist teaching concepts and skills. After the initial learning is in place, the process is expanded to family members and for children, teachers, and other school personnel. This is because NCLT encourages clients to practice new ways of thinking and behavior in everyday life. NCLT is focused on providing the client the tools to understand and operationalize their thoughts, feelings, and emotions.

The ultimate goal is for the client to take over monitoring and modifying the behaviors and thoughts that contribute to their mental health. For young children, this will inevitably mean that the parents are trained in the process so that they may continue to cue their children until the child develops the cognitive sophistication to take over the process.

The Process of Therapy

Therapy is a process of taking previously maladaptive automatic behaviors and thoughts, de-automatizing them and creating new adaptive automatic behaviors and thoughts (responses) to life's various situations. Therapy in this perspective is about the therapist imparting information and having the person use that information to change behavior and emotional response sets. Attaining ultimate success in terms of self-fulfillment or realizing one's potential would be in effect a decision that an individual made when they were no longer engaging in identifiably maladaptive behavior. The practicing therapists and client's job is to select learning opportunities and design activities that will make learning and automatizing adaptive behaviors and thoughts more efficient. Significant others in the person's life are critical in identifying these learning situations. For children this often includes both parents and teachers.

NCLT Is a Model Based on Teaching

All therapy represents a form of learning. There are ways to make learning the material associated with therapeutic change efficient, and there are ways to do it inefficiently. As in other forms of learning, NCLT strives to produce learners who understand how they learn and can use that understanding to continually enhance and develop their knowledge and effectiveness. We teach strategies based upon learning principles.

NCLT Respects What Is Known About the Conduct of a Therapist

The principles that embody NCLT practice are not meant to supplant what is known about the value of the therapeutic relationship. NCLT therapists acknowledge that while the creation of a supportive therapeutic relationship is an important attribute of any therapeutic interaction it, by itself, is not sufficient to insure the effectiveness of the relationship between a therapist and a client. NCLT therapists recognize that liking each other is not the goal of therapy. In fact, while a relationship might be positive, as evidenced by the client's positive regard of the therapist and vice versa, there exists the possibility that, within such a context, the client may in fact not be learning or understanding anything.

Effectiveness is defined in NCLT practice as making measureable progress towards the specific outcomes that were developed at the beginning of treatment. What is most important is that the therapist must understand where in the development of ideas and concepts the client is, so that information can be presented that is accessible and useable by the client. For this to occur, the therapist must understand how certain constructs are developed, and then be able to guide the client on a predictable path to the healthy development of those constructs.

The Core Principles of NCLT

The best way to understand NCLT is to understand its core principles. NCLT really has three sets of principles that govern its operation. By understanding these principles you will have a good deal of insight into what is happening in treatment for your student.

The therapist must focus on the client and how they will incorporate and utilize new knowledge.

It is important to understand that, for a variety of reasons, all information is not useable all the time. There are preconditions that must be met before new information is accessible and usable by the client. Some of these preconditions are as follows:

New Information Must Be at Odds with Existing Information
The process of cognitive and related emotional change is initiated when an individual realizes a new idea does not align with his current thinking or prior knowledge. NCLT posits that for therapy to be successful it is necessary for this moment of conflict to be purposeful, explicit, and clearly expected by the client to occur as part of therapy. In NCLT therapy the client understands that the purposeful challenges to the status quo emotionally and behaviorally will be made. For that to occur, the client must first be cognizant and able to identify the components of a current schema surrounding the construct and recognize that the new idea or fact is discordant with the information already held. NCLT recognizes that when this moment of conflict occurs, an individual will seek out answers in order to align their thinking and resolve the conflict.

New Information Can't Be Too Challenging or It Will Be Rejected
A goal in NCLT treatment is to cause changes in the target concept that to lead to a new understanding and expansion of the concept. Information that is too discordant with the existing information or represents very significant differences between what is known and what is new will represent too difficult a challenge for an individual will be rejected.

New Information Must Be Compared with Existing Information

NCLT recognizes that it is critically important that both the therapist and the client examine the new information in relation to what is known, and discuss how it might be used to impact the target behavior. This is an active and ongoing discussion between therapist and client as the work together to discuss the effect of the new behavior or belief. NCLT therapists understand that most clients, while stating that they desire improvement, really like and wish to hold on to their existing behaviors and beliefs. This is because they have worked hard to learn them and they have become, in many instances, automatic. Leaving the resolution of conflict solely for the client to address increases the probability that the new information may be rejected. In addition, if it does get included, the way that it gets included may be neither what the therapist intended nor desirable. The therapist should of course be aware that in some instances, where beliefs are rigidly held, it is easier for an individual to reject the new information to preserve the core belief.

New Information Is Appended onto Existing Information

New information is not learned snippet by snippet and retained in isolation. Rather, new information is appended onto existing information. This implies that you cannot just add an adaptive response or thought onto what is an already existing body of maladaptive behaviors and thoughts. NCLT recognizes that entire clusters of thoughts related to certain topics and actions will have to be critically challenged and altered.

There is no knowledge independent of the meaning attributed to it by prior experience. Knowledge is constructed by the client.

No information is processed by an individual independently of what that individual already knows. New information is always appended to existing memory in order to be remembered. If the therapist is going to provide information designed to alter a maladaptive belief or set of beliefs (depression), it is necessary to identify for both the therapist and the client how that existing set of beliefs operate and how they distort new information to conform to existing thought patterns.

The examination of how the existing schema encodes information should be the primary task of the intervention, and should occur before the actual attempts at altering are made. Without this information it is possible, and in some instances likely, that those maladaptive beliefs and behaviors will actually be reinforced by the therapeutic intervention.

In therapy it is the client who decides which sensory input is important, to construct meaning out of and commit to memory.

Clients in therapy do not consider everything said during the course of therapy as important or worthy of retention in memory. Listeners actively choose which information to attend to and remember. Changing what clients attend to is more important than what clients actually practice telling themselves. This process of selected attention to specific material, and the ignoring of other material, is termed gating.

Clients, not therapists, ultimately get to determine what is important and what is not, and it is highly possible that clients may select things to attend to that are extraneous to the process of treatment. NCLT therapists understand this process and engage actively with their clients to help them focus on critical areas of the materials to be learned.

The construction of meaning in therapy is a purposeful activity.

Clients construct systematically more advanced and complex adaptive schema (bodies of knowledge). It is the construction of the schema that determines how new knowledge is both interpreted and potentially incorporated. Once learned, clients subconsciously rehearse and refine these new schemas and related strategies to move them towards automaticity.

Automaticity

At the beginning of therapy a client will present with a number of problem behaviors and/or ideas which are causing them difficulty. These behaviors and ideas are the result of a complex and extensive learning history that, through the continuing interaction between existing schema and new information in the environment, produced the current automatic default condition.

Learning in therapy consists both of constructing new meaning and new systems of interrelated meaning. The goal of this learning is to develop a system of adaptive behavior and thought. In most instances this new system of adaptive behavior and thought will be at odds with the existing and entrenched system of maladaptive behavior and thought. In order to make therapeutic progress, the new system of adaptive behavior and thought must be reinforced and encouraged to the point of automaticity, while the existing maladaptive schema must be made nonautomatic. This is a two pronged process. The new adaptive system must be purposefully selected and practiced in many environments while at the same time the old maladaptive system must be purposefully deselected and not practiced in those same environments.

All of this requires precision in definition and in identifying therapeutic behavioral and emotional outcomes. It also requires that the client to understand and participate in the process of constructing new and adaptive schema.

New Behaviors Are Clumsy

Treatment will initially produce a new response schema that is poorly developed, skeletal, poorly generalized, and poorly interconnected. This means that the client will likely not spontaneously use the new information outside of the therapeutic environment. This new schema must be purposefully developed and practiced to the point of automaticity. The client must be an active participant in this process. The process is best accomplished with clearly defined learning outcomes and specific teaching strategies designed to reach those outcomes. Individuals learn better and develop efficient subconscious rehearsal strategies when goals are clearly articulated.

Humans learn by pattern matching. Each meaning we construct makes us better able to give meaning to other stimuli which can match with a previously identified and categorized, similar pattern.

When we encounter a new stimulus, the brain immediately begins to attempt to match it with what is already known. Humans pattern match between crucial issues in the environment and elements of mental schemata to determine which schemata will be accessed and used to append the new information. Classes of stimuli are grouped together in the brain. Clients seeking treatment often have whole classes of stimuli (schemata) that they react poorly to.

On occasion, increasing exposure and information can amend a schema or split it into two related schemata. Suppose, for example, you were afraid of all spiders and reacted with a great deal of anxiety to an appearance of any spider. Now suppose you were motivated by your new job at the arachnoid exhibit at the zoo and took the time to learn about spiders and found out which ones were dangerous and which were not. Eventually you would develop two highly related schemata, spiders which were dangerous and spiders which were not. The response patterns to these schemata would be different. NCLT therapy works in a similar fashion. The goal of treatment is to make the response patterns of individual's to specific schema explicit so that they can be examined and modified. Maladaptive responses should be deconditioned, and adaptive responses practiced and automatized.

The construction of meaning is neurophysiologically based and involves brain circuitry dedicated to pattern matching, learning, and reinforcement recognition.

All information that is learned is processed over the same neural networks. There is no separate system for material learned in therapy, although there may be, as a result of the emotional valence of the material, different brain regions recruited for specific elements of what is discussed in treatment.

Specific recruitment of brain regions is not unique to learning in a therapeutic context, it is a characteristic of all learning. Regions responsible for emotional valence and reward recognition are not the exclusive domain of the material learned in therapy. These regions are recruited by any activity which is accompanied by a level of arousal. The regions which are responsible for reward recognition are critical in the gating process. Gating is the process that determines what information is accepted into working memory, and therefore determines what material is available to be worked on in therapy.

Therapists knowingly or unknowingly provide encouragement, direction, and support.

Clearly the degree to which the relationship between the therapist and the client produces an environment for encouragement and support is a factor in determining the effect of therapy. It is clear that the therapists' approval and support is as source of reinforcement that is used by all therapists to guide and shape the course of learning.

The language we use influences learning. Language and learning are inextricably intertwined.

Language is a critical tool for the shaping and reshaping of thought and related emotional states. The directed, purposeful, and structured use of language is important for imparting information designed to change cognition. Obviously, the haphazard or inefficient use of this tool would produce less than optimal results. Therefore, those systems that make purposeful use of language are to be preferred to less directed systems where the expected impact of language is not planned, or in fact the use of language itself, is minimized.

Learning in therapy is a social activity. To be useful, knowledge acquired in therapy must be applied and practiced within the context of both new and existing relationships.

There are two separate points here, the first of which is that learning is a social process with at least two active participants, and the second is that new learning must be practiced in those social contexts in which it was intended. This practice must be purposeful and directed. New behavior must be practiced in the social world for it to be incorporated into the automatic repertoire of the learner. Such practice represents the core of a planned and purposeful therapy process. The learning outcome for the practice should be known to the learner so that the result of the practice can be integrated into the appropriate body of existing knowledge. The goal is automaticity of new behavior into the repertoire of the individual.

Learning in therapy is contextual. We learn in relationship to what else we already know, and what we already believe.

Just as in building academic skill sets, a sound foundation is necessary. In therapy it is not desirable to append adaptive knowledge to maladaptive preexisting knowledge. To be effective, new skill sets and their associated cognitions must be developed and practiced. In practice, this is difficult to do because humans show a strong tendency to hold onto prior knowledge and discount new knowledge that is not in agreement with prior knowledge. In other words, if the new knowledge disagrees with what I already believe, I have a strong tendency to reject the new knowledge to protect my existing beliefs. Indeed, it can be argued that one purpose of knowledge is to develop attitudes and belief systems that are resistant to change, and that this rejection of new beliefs or knowledge serves a valuable protective function.

In order to understand how this process works, it is important to know that as we have discussed, humans learn by pattern matching. When we first encounter a novel stimulus we search what we know, looking for similar patterns or constructs to relate it to. We then look at this information in light of what we already know. We can do one of three basic things with this new knowledge. We can accept it and alter what we already know. We can reject it and protect what we already know. Or we can consider it, and see how it fits in with what we already know.

As we have seen, humans have a propensity to protect what we already know and therefore, the most likely scenario when confronted with new information is to reject it outright. The second most likely event is to consider it, and see how it fits in with what we already know, and the least likely outcome is to accept the discordant new information and throw away, or irrevocably alter what we already know. Much of what the lay person thinks about when they think about therapy is defined by this last most unlikely outcome. People believe that the therapist will say something, and on the basis of that statement, a transformation of the maladaptive body of knowledge will occur. As we have just learned, this is both unlikely and counter to the actual tendency of people when they encounter new information.

What is more likely, and in fact therapeutically desirable, is that the client (learner) engages in the middle option. They will use the new information to see how it relates to what they already know. You may know this as critical thinking. We do know a few things about how this occurs. One of the most important things is that for this objective analysis to occur, the learner must be motivated to do the comparison, and dispassionate about the analysis. The stronger the attitude is held, the more difficult the comparison is to make. In addition, beliefs associated with strong affect states lead to strongly held attitudes which are more resistant to change.

All of this goes to the point that in order to change the strongly held, emotionally laden belief systems that characterize the thinking of people with emotional problems, the clients must be encouraged to do a systematic and dispassionate analysis of those belief systems in an environment or in a manner that does not threaten the client and cause the client to withdraw. New information must be presented that is just different enough and minimally threatening enough to enable the client to process it, while at the same time be both novel and interesting enough to encourage the allocation of working memory to the process. This calls for a careful and thoughtful assessment of the type of new information, its purpose, and how it will be offered to the client. This argues persuasively that clients should not be left to their own devices to filter the information provided in a therapeutic exchange because their natural tendency will be to reject new information or avoid comparison or questioning their passionately held attitudes. The job of the therapist is, with the learning outcome clearly in mind, to systematically prepare the stimuli so that they meet the just right challenge and create an environment wherein the client is open to and engaged in confronting maladaptive attitudes and beliefs. By a process of shaping and desensitization, the therapist should present new information designed to challenge the existing attitude while at the same time not being threatening to it.

It is not possible to assimilate new knowledge without having some structure developed from previous knowledge upon which to build.

Learning is incremental. The more we know, the more we can learn. Therefore, any effort to teach must be connected to the state of the client, and must provide a clear, direct, and unambiguous path into the subject for the learner that emanates from the learner's (client's) previous knowledge. This implies that adaptive beliefs and constructs should form the basis of new learning, and that therapy should be directed towards both creating the functional beliefs, attitudes, and skill sets and then practicing those skill sets in multiple environments.

Learning occurs when some responses are trained and selected, and others are not trained and are deselected. Learning is effective when this process is directed and specific, with the learning paths specified and reinforced. Learning is then enhanced through a process of refinement of, and automization of, these selected responses.

Learning new ideas and ways of behaving in therapy is not instantaneous.

Learning requires both practice and rewards. Clients must recognize old ideas as maladaptive, and actively seek to replace them with new ideas based upon a foundation of new learning and successful application. Research has suggested that learning new skills or changing existing cognitive schema is enhanced, in terms of increased automaticity, when new concepts are pulled into working memory and then used in multiple applications. In order to create these various applications, guided practice enhanced with behavioral practice improves learning efficiency. To effect learning and generalization of new constructs in therapy, highly structured and guided instruction is necessary to create the new schema. Only after the new schema is constructed it is beneficial to reduce guidance and structure.

Motivation is a key component in learning. Not only is it the case that motivation helps learning, it is essential for learning.

For NCLT, motivation is not the product of a mystical personality trait that certain individuals either have in abundance or in which they are deficit. For NCLT, motivation reflects the operation of the reward recognition circuit which is either more or less efficiently integrated with behavioral circuits. Success is reinforcing and results in the increased likelihood the action will continue to be selected in the future. Therapeutic progress therefore is facilitated when a planned program of increasingly complex actions is engaged in and reinforced. Motivation is therefore derived from successful practice and automatization of target behaviors designed to achieve a specific goal.

Maladaptive behavior and thought is based upon automaticity.

Automaticity is the goal of human learning. In this regard maladaptive thought and resulting behavior is no different than any other type of thought including adaptive thought. It is learned in the same way, expressed behaviorally in the same way, and automatized in the same way. The neural circuitry involved in its learning is the same neural circuitry that is involved in all other learning, including math and reading. From this we can conclude that the neural circuitry over which the maladaptive learning took place is functioning entirely appropriately. It is only that the learned connections lead to less than adaptive behavior and thought. Therefore, brains are not defectively permanently wired, or permanently damaged. It is not guaranteed that a person with an emotional dysregulation issue has a badly wired brain. In many instances the diagnosis merely implies that the current patterns of connectivity are the result of reinforcement patterns that have not produced adaptive behavior. NCLT posits that, in most instances, this is not a permanent condition. These pathways supporting maladaptive behavior can be altered by the same processes that supported their formation in the first place.

The ability to solve problems and the ability to adapt to novel situations are positively correlated with improved mental health.

Learning occurs when potential responses to environmental occurrences are reweighted with some responses being made more likely and other responses becoming less likely.

Both working memory and processing speed efficiency play important roles in this process. Deselection and reselection depends on the ability to suppress (deselect) newly identified task-irrelevant information as well as the ability to activate (select) newly identified task-relevant information. Efficient working memory results in material being held in working memory for a greater period of time and being increasingly available for modification. This leads to the potential for increased flexibility which in turn implies increased ability to evaluate novel solutions and consider new responses. It also suggests increased ability to select a new response to make automatic.

Therapy is cognitively demanding.

Deselection and reselection of a new process to make automatic (the process of therapy) is at first a conscious, planned, and time-consuming process. An individual who is attempting to eliminate a maladaptive, automatized process such as a complex maladaptive behavioral response or thought will struggle due to the required cognitive effort. It is likely that they will become even more inefficient and ineffective as they shift from their maladaptive strategies to newer, potentially effective but not yet automatic cognitive processes. Support here becomes critical.

Learning is about connections in that what is stored together stays together in memory.

Learning new things in therapy, as in all other learning, occurs in context. What is learned is associated and remembered in the context of what was around it during the time it was encountered. Therefore, it is critical to the process of therapy that newly learned adaptive responses should be practiced in as many new contexts as is possible. This practice should be a planned and purposeful part of treatment and not just be left to circumstance.

The basic principles of learning for NCLT are:

1. Learning is a product of working memory allocation
2. Working memory's capacity for allocation is affected by prior knowledge
3. Working memory allocation is directed by motivation

NCLT offers the following as rules that govern the process of knowledge acquisition in therapy.

If knowledge in long-term memory is retrieved, the strength of association between all items retrieved to working memory is increased. Clinically this implies that how things are presented and grouped in working memory determines what procedures will be developed from their association.

If a knowledge is retrieved, all other elements of knowledge to which it is connected are retrieved, and all connections are strengthened.

If parts of retrieved knowledge match to working memory contents, the connection between the existing knowledge and the new material are strengthened. If parts of retrieved knowledge do not match to contents in working memory, the connections are weakened and inhibited. Establishing new pattern matches (schemata) is an essential component in therapy.

If an action is successful, its connection to the knowledge of the situation in which it occurred is strengthened. If an action is unsuccessful, its connection to the knowledge of the situation in which it occurred is weakened or inhibited. The therapeutic implication of this is that new procedures must be understood and conscientiously practiced.

If knowledge has been retrieved, new information in working memory will be connected to this knowledge. This is the basis of establishing new adaptive procedures.

Any active knowledge in long-term memory is accessible to working memory.

The Goal of Therapy Is Also Competence

The term competence has been used to refer to accumulated learning experiences that result in a pattern of effective adaptation within an environment. Within the NCLT clinical context, it implies that the individual has (or lacking competence does not have) the capability to perform well in the future. Like many cognitive therapy models NCLT posits that an individual who lacks competence in an environment becomes self-aware and engages in negative self-appraisals. These negative self-appraisals are reinforced and reproduced regularly until they are automatically associated with a class of behaviors or physiological responses. NCLT theory hypothesizes that these automatically associated physiological responses and appraisals are experienced as affect states such as depression and anxiety. That is, in part, because the physiological responses associated with these affect states are also associated through the same principles of learning, to the cognitions associated with the appraisals.

Summary

The astute educator will probably recognize that many of the above principles are identical to those that govern knowledge acquisition in the classroom and that is, of course, exactly the point. All therapy is about learning. For children, educators have an important role in this process, and must be intensively involved in the identification and creation of new and adaptive learning targets.

Appendix B: Parent Orientation to Neurocognitive Learning Therapy

You and your child are about to start a planned learning experience designed to teach your child new and more adaptive ways to handle the stressors and behavioral difficulties that have proved challenging in the past. Although the primary target of this treatment is your child, it is important to know that the entire family will have to participate for the treatment is to be successful. You are vitally important in this process. This guide is designed to provide you with important information about what is going to be occurring in treatment. In addition, it will provide information designed to help you to know how to support your child's treatment at home.

Please make sure you work with your child's therapist to establish the goals and objectives for treatment, and identify the learning situations that happen at home that provide opportunities for your child to practice their new behavior. If you have questions after you have finished reviewing this guide, please make sure you schedule time to get the answers you need.

What Is Neurocognitive Learning Therapy?

Neurocognitive learning therapy (NCLT) is a therapeutic system designed to work with and make use of our understanding of how the human brain processes and learns information. For NCLT, therapy is considered a process of increasing the likelihood of the expression of adaptive behaviors, healthy emotional responding and thought processes, and weakening or unlearning maladaptive ones. For NCLT, the therapy process goal is to eliminate maladaptive behaviors and thoughts which have become automatic, and develop new, adaptive behaviors and thoughts which will become automatic. NCLT represents a fusion of information processing theory, brain network models and cognitive behavioral treatment models, within a developmental perspective. It comes from the perspective of mental health, teaching new ways to have healthier thoughts, feelings, and behavioral expressions. It has a strong respect for the developmental level of the person we work with, and where in the life course they currently are.

What Is the Neurophysiological Basis of NCLT?

A basic premise of NCLT is that all learning begins at birth. Learning both affects, and is affected by, the developing brain and the interaction with the environment. Whatever the subject, issue or person and emotional valence thereof, learning occurs over the same neural networks, and is subject to the same laws governing working memory allocation, attention, processing efficiency, memory, expression, and engagement. The goal of therapy is to learn healthy, adaptive behaviors, emotions, and patterns. Therapy for younger children also includes the benefit of preventing the patterning or learning of maladaptive patterns.

All environmental experiences provide the opportunity to learn adaptive behavior. Sometimes, however, we don't. Understanding this makes it possible to develop a set of principles that would facilitate learning within the therapeutic environment. The experiences we provide in therapy to facilitate learning are designed to provide the opportunity to unlearn maladaptive behavioral or emotional responses to various environmental exigencies, and learn more adaptive behaviors and emotional responses. How this expedited learning occurs in an environment where an individual is seeking to address issues related to mental health (therapy) is at the core of NCLT.

NCLT Is a Unique System

NCLT is not a type of therapy. It is a system of therapy. NCLT does not fall neatly into any of the existing therapeutic disciplines that you might be familiar with. The therapeutic principles that form the core of NCLT actually underlie the functionality of every other therapeutic modality. As such, it represents the common core of all therapeutic techniques. This permits and supports the use of many other therapeutic techniques within NCLT practice. Rather than a therapeutic model with a single focus, NCLT is more of a broad educational experience; The concepts, principles, and skills that are central to NCLT are taught to individuals. The client, irrespective of their age, becomes an active participant.

The Basics of NCLT

The Principle of Memory Reconciliation

Recently, three independent groups of researchers using specific therapeutic techniques utilized in NCLT have demonstrated the ability to activate a learned emotional response, and under certain conditions found that its previously locked neural circuit had temporarily shifted back into an unlocked, de-consolidated, labile, destabilized, or plastic state. This unlocked state allowed prior maladaptive learning to be completely unlearned, along with behavioral responses it had been driving. The temporarily labile circuit soon consolidates once again, returning to a locked condition. The researchers named this newly discovered type of neuroplasticity "memory reconsolidation."

Prior to this research, the prevailing wisdom was that learning that had occurred in the presence of a strong emotion became locked permanently into subcortical implicit memory circuits by special synapses, never to be unlocked. They were permanently wired and would always be evoked when some trigger occurred. This implied that people had to accept that they could never change the way that they react to things, that they just had to get used to it, and adjust accordingly. Fortunately, this wisdom was wrong.

Research has identified a number of clinical conditions whose symptomology is alleviated by memory reconsolidation that occurs as part of NCLT (Table A.1).

This new knowledge forms the neuropsychological and neurophysiological basis for NCLT. Clinically, this means that while physiological responses may be hard

Table A.1 Disorders whose symptomology are alleviated by memory reconsolidation

Attention deficit/hyperactivity disorder	Anxiety	Anger
Attachment disorder	Compulsive behavior	Depression
Guilt	Low arousal	Low motivation
Low self-worth	Poor motivation	Posttraumatic stress disorder
Perfectionism	Panic attacks	Phobic responses

wired, counteracting and regulating unwanted acquired responses are not the way to resolve emotional issues. Rather, relearning or learning the adaptive response is.

NCLT is designed to (re)teach adaptive emotional responses using well-established principles of learning, working in conjunction with specific empirically valid therapeutic techniques.

Memory Reconsolidation in Therapy

In order for the memories that trigger the maladaptive emotional response to be unlearned, a critical experience must take place in therapy. In order to accomplish this, the emotional memory and related maladaptive behavioral response is first reactivated. This critical experience should provide perceptions that sharply mismatch or deviate substantially from what the reactivated target memory expects, and predicts about how the world functions. This is what happens in therapy. Clinically, the mismatch can be either a full contradiction or disconfirmation of the target memory or a novel, salient variation relative to the target memory. If the target memory is reactivated by familiar cues, but not concurrently mismatched, synapses do not unlock and reconsolidation is not induced.

A three-step process is initially required in order to carry out the sequence eliminating the maladaptive memory and program a new adaptive memory and related behavior.

- Symptom identification. Actively clarify with the client what to regard as the presenting symptom(s). These include the specific behaviors, somatics, emotions, and/or thoughts that the client wants to eliminate and when they happen.
- Retrieval of target learning into explicit awareness, as a visceral emotional experience, the details of the emotional learning underlying and driving the presenting symptom.
- Identification of disconfirming knowledge. Identify a vivid experience (past or present) that can serve as living knowledge that is fundamentally incompatible with the model of reality in the target emotional learning retrieved in the prior step, such that both cannot possibly be true. The disconfirming material may or may not be appealing to the client as being more "positive" or preferred; what matters is that it be mutually exclusive with the target learning. It may be already part of the client's personal knowledge or may be created by a new experience.

There is a fourth step wherein the client verifies the new emotional response by generalizing it into new situations and contexts.

Reward Recognition

Estimates vary but it has been suggested that human adults make 35,000 remotely conscious decisions each day. Assuming 16 waking hours each day that's almost 2200 decisions every hour, 36 decisions every minute, and 1 decision about every second and a half. Young children make as few as 3000 decisions in a day. Decisions represent choices between two or more options. That's what your child is doing when they choose between doing their homework and playing their favorite video game. They are making a choice between two options. These decisions are not isolated instances. Each one builds upon the other. These compounded choices not only build upon each other, they act interdependently with other contextually relevant decisions resulting in a complex web of interconnected patterns of actions and emotional responses.

Some decisions are practiced so much that they become automatic; we do them without having to think about them. After some practice we no longer think about them individually, they automatically occur in a sequence.

NCLT teaches that when a person is confronted by making a choice between two or more stimuli a separate sampling process for each attribute of each of the available choices is conducted. When we are thinking about deciding between choices our attention switches from one attribute consideration to the next. The order in which attributes are considered as well for how long each attribute is considered (attention time) influences the predicted choice probabilities and choice response times. Both order of attribute consideration and attention time given to each attribute are important targets for discussion within an NCLT session.

Perceived rewards are critical part of the consideration of choice attributes. For NCLT, understanding the value of rewarding and punishing stimuli from your child's perspective will enable an understanding of when and where such rewards and punishments will be identified and used. Helping your child identify potentially rewarding aspects of the desirable choice you wish them to make is an important part of the work in NCLT.

The Role of the Parent

Parents can be valuable in this process because they can help identify many of the targets to practice as well as many of the disconfirming events. They can identify maladaptive responses (emotional or behavioral) that are causing their child difficulty. Then working in conjunction with the NCLT therapist, they can help by recognizing situations at home that call for the newly taught adaptive response and cuing the child to engage in it. Parents can also point out the inconsistencies between the original perception and the realities at home. Many times in therapy situations that produce maladaptive responses can only be discussed because the situations arise in the child's everyday life outside of the therapy environment. Parents are uniquely qualified to both identify these events and to support the elimination of maladaptive responses and the relearning of adaptive ones by cuing those adaptive responses to occur.

What Happens in Therapy?

NCLT Is About Learning

From an NCLT perspective, a therapist assumes an active, instructive, and authoritative role, and teaches patients to think and conduct themselves differently. This is initially a collaboration between the therapist and the client with the therapist teaching concepts and skills. After the initial learning is in place, the process is expanded to family members and, for children, teachers, and other school personnel. This is because NCLT encourages clients to practice new ways of thinking and behaviors in everyday life. NCLT is focused on providing the client the tools to understand and operationalize their thoughts, feelings, and emotions.

The ultimate goal is for the client to take over monitoring and modifying the behaviors and thoughts that contribute to their mental health. For young children, this will inevitably mean that the parents are trained in the process so that they may continue to cue their children until the child develops the cognitive sophistication to take over the process themselves.

The Process of Therapy

Therapy is a process of taking previously maladaptive, automatic behaviors and thoughts, de-automatizing them and creating new adaptive automatic behaviors and thoughts (responses) to life's various situations. Therapy in this perspective is about the therapist imparting information and having the person use that information to change behavior and emotional response sets. Attaining ultimate success in terms of self-fulfillment or realizing one's potential would be in effect a decision that an individual made when they were no longer engaging in identifiably maladaptive behavior. The practicing therapists and clients job is to select learning opportunities and design activities that will make learning and automatizing adaptive behaviors and thoughts more efficient. Significant others in the person's life are critical in identifying these learning situations. For children, this often includes both parents and teachers.

NCLT Is a Model Based on Teaching

All therapy represents a form of learning. As in other forms of learning, NCLT strives to produce learners who understand how they learn so that they can use that understanding to continually enhance and develop their knowledge and effectiveness. We teach strategies based upon learning principles with the intent of our clients being able to take that information and continue to correctly apply it on their own.

NCLT Respects What Is Known About the Conduct of a Therapist

NCLT therapists acknowledge that while the creation of a supportive therapeutic relationship is an important attribute of any therapeutic interaction it, by itself, is not sufficient to insure the effectiveness of the relationship between a therapist and a client. NCLT therapists recognize that liking each other is not the goal of therapy. In fact, while a relationship might be positive, as evidenced by the clients positive regard of the therapist and vice versa, there exists the possibility that, within such a context, the client may in fact not be learning or understanding anything.

Effectiveness is defined in NCLT practice as making measureable progress towards the specific outcomes that were developed at the beginning of treatment. What is most important is that the therapist must understand where in the development of ideas and concepts your child is so that information can be presented that is accessible, and useable. For this to occur, the therapist must understand how certain constructs are developed, and then be able to guide the client on a predictable path to the healthy development of those constructs.

The Core Principles of NCLT

The best way to understand NCLT is to understand its core principles. NCLT really has three sets of principles that govern its operation. By understanding these principles you will have a good deal of insight into what is happening in treatment for your child.

The therapist must focus on the client and how they will incorporate and utilize new knowledge.
It is important to understand that, for a variety of reasons, all information is not useable all the time. There are preconditions that must be met before new information is accessible and usable by the client. Some of these preconditions are as follows:

New Information Must Be at Odds with Existing Information
The process of cognitive and related emotional change is initiated when an individual realizes a new idea does not align with his current thinking or prior knowledge. NCLT posits that for therapy to be successful, it is necessary for this moment of conflict to be purposeful, explicit, and clearly expected by the client to occur as part of therapy. In NCLT therapy, the client understands that the purposeful challenges to the status quo emotionally and behaviorally will be made. For that to occur the client must first be cognizant and able to identify the components of a current schema surrounding the construct and recognize that the new idea or fact is discordant with the information already held. NCLT recognizes that when this moment of conflict occurs, an individual will seek out answers in order to align their thinking and resolve the conflict.

New Information Can't Be Too Challenging or It Will Be Rejected
A goal in NCLT treatment is to cause changes in the target concept that to lead to a new understanding and expansion of the concept. Information that is too discordant with the existing information or represents very significant differences between what is known and what is new will represent too difficult a challenge for an individual will be rejected.

New Information Must Be Compared with Existing Information
NCLT recognizes that it is critically important that both the therapist and the client examine the new information in relation to what is known, and discuss how it might be used to impact the target behavior. This is an active and ongoing discussion between therapist and client as the work together to discuss the effect of the new behavior or belief. NCLT therapists understand that most clients, while stating that they desire improvement, really like and wish to hold on to their existing behaviors and beliefs. This is because they have worked hard to learn them and they are in many instances automatic. Leaving the resolution of conflict solely for the client to do increases the probability that the new information may be rejected. In addition, if it does get included the way that it gets included may be neither what the therapist intended nor desirable. The therapist should of course be aware that in some instances, where beliefs are rigidly held, it is easier for an individual to reject the new information to preserve the core belief.

New Information Is Appended onto Existing Information

New information is not learned snippet by snippet and retained in isolation. New information is appended onto existing information. This implies that you cannot just add an adaptive response or thought onto what is an already existing body of maladaptive behaviors and thoughts. NCLT recognizes that entire clusters of thoughts related to certain topic and actions will have to be critically challenged and altered.

There is no knowledge independent of the meaning attributed to it by prior experience. Knowledge is constructed by the client.

No information is processed by an individual independently of what that individual already knows. New information is always appended to existing memory in order to be remembered. If the therapist is going to provide information designed to alter a maladaptive belief or set of beliefs (depression), it is necessary to identify for both the therapist and the client how that existing set of beliefs operate and how they distort new information to conform to existing thought patterns.

The examination of how the existing schema encodes information should be the primary task of the intervention and should occur before the actual attempts at altering are made. Without this information it is possible, and in some instances likely, that those maladaptive beliefs and behaviors will actually be reinforced by the therapeutic intervention.

In therapy it is the child who decides which sensory input is important, to construct meaning out of and commit to memory.

Children in therapy do not consider everything said during the course of therapy as important or worthy of retention in memory. Listeners actively choose which information to attend to and remember. Changing what clients attend to is more important than what clients actually practice telling themselves. This process of selected attention to specific material, and the ignoring of other material, is termed gating.

Children, not therapists, ultimately get to determine what is important and what is not, and it is highly possible that they may select things to attend to that are extraneous to the process of treatment. NCLT therapists understand this process and engage actively with their clients to help them focus on critical areas of the materials to be learned.

The construction of meaning in therapy is a purposeful activity.

Clients construct systematically more advanced and complex adaptive schema (bodies of knowledge). It is the construction of the schema that determines how new knowledge is both interpreted and potentially incorporated. Once learned, clients subconsciously rehearse and refine these new schemas and related strategies to move them towards automaticity.

Automaticity

At the beginning of therapy a client will present with a number of problem behaviors and/or ideas which are causing them difficulty. These behaviors and ideas are the result of a complex and extensive learning history that, through the continuing interaction between existing schema and new information in the environment, produced the current automatic default condition.

Learning in therapy consists both of constructing new meaning and new systems of interrelated meaning. The goal of this learning is to develop a system of adaptive behavior and thought. In most instances this new system of adaptive behavior and thought will be at odds with the existing and entrenched system of maladaptive behavior and thought. In order to make therapeutic progress the new system of adaptive behavior and thought must be reinforced and encouraged to the point of automaticity while the existing maladaptive schema must be made nonautomatic. This is a two pronged process. The new adaptive system must be purposefully selected and practiced in many environments while at the same time the old mal-adaptive system must be purposefully deselected and not practiced in those same environments.

New Behaviors Are Unstable

Treatment will, initially, produce a new response schema that is poorly developed, skeletal, poorly generalized, and poorly interconnected. This means that the client will likely not spontaneously use the new information outside of the therapeutic environment. This new schema must be purposefully developed and practiced to the point of automaticity. The client must be an active participant in this process. The process is best accomplished with clearly defined learning outcomes and specific teaching strategies designed to reach those outcomes. Individuals learn better and develop efficient, subconscious rehearsal strategies when goals are clearly articulated.

Humans learn by pattern matching. Each meaning we construct makes us better able to give meaning to other stimuli which can match with a previously identified and categorized, similar pattern.

When we encounter a new stimuli the brain immediately begins to attempt to match it with what is already known. Humans pattern match between crucial issues in the environment and elements of mental schemata to determine which schemata will be accessed and used to append the new information. Classes of stimuli are grouped together in the brain. Clients seeking treatment often have whole classes of stimuli (schemata) that they react poorly to.

On occasion, increasing exposure and information can amend a schema or split it into two related schemata. Suppose, for example, you were afraid of all spiders and reacted with a great deal of anxiety to an appearance of any spider. Now suppose you were motivated by your new job at the arachnoid exhibit at the zoo and took the time to learn about spiders and found out which ones were dangerous and which were not. Eventually you would develop two highly related schemata, spiders which were dangerous and spiders which were not. The response patterns to these schemata would be different. NCLT therapy works in a similar fashion. The goal of treatment is to make the response patterns of individual's to specific schema explicit so that they can be examined and modified. Maladaptive responses should be deconditioned, and adaptive responses practiced and automatized.

The construction of meaning is neurophysiologically based and involves brain circuitry dedicated to pattern matching, learning, and reinforcement recognition.

All information that is learned is processed over the same neural networks. There is no separate system for material learned in therapy, although there may be, as a result of the emotional valence of the material, different brain regions recruited for specific elements of what is discussed in treatment.

Specific recruitment of brain regions is not unique to learning in a therapeutic context, it is a characteristic of all learning. Regions responsible for emotional valence and reward recognition are not the exclusive domain of the material learned in therapy. These regions are recruited by any activity which is accompanied by a level of arousal. The regions which are responsible for reward recognition are critical in the gating process. Gating is the process that determines what information is accepted into working memory and therefore determines what material is available to be worked on in therapy.

Therapists knowingly or unknowingly provide encouragement, direction, and support.

Clearly the degree to which the relationship between the therapist and the client produces an environment for encouragement and support is a factor in determining the effect of therapy. It is clear that the therapists' approval and support is as source of reinforcement that is used by all therapists to guide and shape the course of learning.

The language we use influences learning. Language and learning are inextricably intertwined.

Language is a critical tool for the shaping and reshaping of thought and related emotional states. The directed, purposeful, and structured use of language is important for imparting information designed to change cognition. Obviously, the haphazard or inefficient use of this tool would produce less than optimal results. Therefore, those systems that make purposeful use of language are to be preferred to less directed systems where the expected impact of language is not planned, or in fact the use of language itself is minimalized.

Learning in therapy is a social activity. To be useful, knowledge acquired in therapy must be applied and practiced within the context of both new and existing relationships.

There are two separate points here, the first of which is that learning is a social process with at least two active participants, and the second is that new learning must be practiced in those social contexts that it was intended to be used in. This practice must be purposeful and directed. New behavior must be practiced in the social world for it to be incorporated into the automatic repertoire of the learner. Such practice represents the core of a planned and purposeful therapy process. The learning outcome for the practice should be known to the learner so that the result of the practice can be integrated into the appropriate body of existing knowledge. The goal is automaticity of new and adaptive behavior into the repertoire of the individual.

Learning in therapy is contextual. We learn in relationship to what else we already know and what we already believe.

In therapy it is not desirable to append adaptive knowledge to maladaptive preexisting knowledge. To be effective, new skill sets and their associated cognitions must be developed and practiced. In practice, this is difficult to do because humans show a strong tendency to hold onto prior knowledge and discount new knowledge that is not in agreement with prior knowledge. In other words, if the new knowledge disagrees with what I already know, I have a strong tendency to reject the new knowledge to protect my existing beliefs. Indeed, it can be argued that one purpose of knowledge is to develop attitudes and belief systems that are resistant to change, and that this rejection of new knowledge serves a valuable protective function.

In order to understand how this process works it is important to know that, as we have discussed, humans learn by pattern matching. When we first encounter a novel stimuli we search what we know, looking for similar patterns or constructs to relate it to. We then look at this information in light of what we already know. We can do of three basic things with this new knowledge. We can accept it and alter what we already know. We can reject it and protect what we already know. Or we can consider it and see how it fits in with what we already know.

As we have seen, humans have a propensity to protect what we already know and therefore, the most likely scenario when confronted with new information is to reject it outright. The second most likely event is to consider it, and see how it fits in with what we already know, and the least likely outcome is to accept the discordant new information and throw away, or irrevocably alter what we already know. Much of what the lay person thinks about when they think about therapy is defined by this last most unlikely outcome. People believe that the therapist will say something, and on the basis of that statement, a transformation of the maladaptive body of knowledge will occur. As we have just learned, this is both unlikely and counter to the actual tendency of people when they encounter new information.

What is more likely, and in fact therapeutically desirable, is that the client (learner) engages in the middle option. They will use the new information to see how it relates to what they already know. We do know a few things about how this occurs. One of the most important things is that for this objective analysis to occur, the learner must be motivated to do the comparison, and dispassionate about the analysis. The stronger the attitude is held, the more difficult the comparison is to make. In addition, beliefs associated with strong affect states lead to strongly held attitudes which are more resistant to change.

All of this goes to the point that in order to change the strongly held, emotionally laden belief systems that characterize the thinking of children with emotional problems, the children must be encouraged to do a systematic and dispassionate analysis of those belief systems in an environment or in a manner that does not threaten the child and cause the child to withdraw. New information must be just different enough and minimally threatening enough to enable the client to process it while at the same time be both novel and interesting enough to encourage the allocation of working memory. This calls for a careful and thoughtful assessment of the type of new information, its purpose, and how it will be offered to the child. This argues persuasively that children should not be left to their own devices to filter the information provided in a therapeutic exchange, because their natural tendency will be to reject new information, or avoid comparison or questioning their passionately held attitudes.

The job of the therapist is, with the learning outcome clearly in mind, to systematically prepare the stimuli so that they meet the just right challenge and create an environment wherein the client is open to and engaged in confronting maladaptive attitudes and beliefs. By a process of shaping and desensitization, the therapist should present new information designed to challenge the existing attitude while at the same time not being threatening to it.

It is not possible to assimilate new knowledge without having some structure developed from previous knowledge upon which to build.

Learning is incremental, the more we know, the more we can learn. Therefore, any effort to teach must be connected to the state of the client, and must provide a clear, direct, and unambiguous path into the subject for the learner that emanates from the learner's (client's) previous knowledge. This implies that adaptive beliefs and constructs should form the basis of new learning, and that therapy should be directed towards both creating the functional beliefs, attitudes, and skill sets and then practicing those skill sets in multiple environments.

Learning occurs when some responses are trained and selected, and others are not trained and are deselected. Learning is effective when this process is directed and specific, with the learning paths specified and reinforced. Learning is then enhanced through a process of refinement of, and automization of, these selected responses.

Learning new ideas and ways of behaving in therapy is not instantaneous.

Learning requires both practice and rewards. Clients must recognize old ideas as maladaptive, and actively seek to replace them with new ideas based upon a foundation of new learning and successful application. Research has suggested that learning new skills or changing existing cognitive schema is enhanced, in terms of increased automaticity, when new concepts are pulled into working memory and then used in multiple applications. In order to create these various applications, guided practice enhanced with behavioral practice improves learning efficiency. To effect learning and generalization of new constructs in therapy, highly structured and guided instruction is necessary to create the new schema. Only after the new schema is constructed it is beneficial to reduce guidance and structure.

Motivation is a key component in learning. Not only is it the case that motivation helps learning, it is essential for learning.

For NCLT, motivation is not the product of a mystical personality trait that certain individuals either have in abundance or in which they are deficit. For NCLT, motivation reflects the operation of the reward recognition circuit which is either more or less efficiently integrated with behavioral circuits. Success brings reinforcement and the increased likelihood the action will continue to be selected in the future. Therapeutic progress therefore is facilitated when a planned program of increasingly complex actions is engaged in and reinforced. Motivation is therefore derived from successful practice and automatization of target behaviors designed to achieve a specific goal.

Maladaptive behavior and thought is based upon automaticity.

Automaticity is the goal of human learning. In this regard maladaptive thought and resulting behavior is no different than any other type of thought including adaptive thought. It is learned in the same way, expressed behaviorally in the same way, and automatized in the same way. The neural circuitry involved in its learning is the same neural circuitry that is involved in all other learning. From this we can conclude that the neural circuitry over which the maladaptive learning took place is functioning entirely appropriately. It is only that the learned connections lead to less than adaptive behavior and thought. Therefore, brains are not defectively permanently wired, or permanently damaged. It is not guaranteed that a person with an emotional dysregulation issue has a badly wired brain. In many instances a diagnosis merely implies that the current patterns of connectivity are the result of reinforcement patterns that have not produced adaptive behavior. NCLT posits that, in most instances, this is not a permanent condition. These pathways supporting maladaptive behavior can be altered by the same processes that supported their formation in the first place.

The ability to solve problems and the ability to adapt to novel situations are positively correlated with improved mental health.

Learning occurs when potential responses to environmental occurrences are reweighted with some responses being made more likely and other responses becoming less likely.

Both working memory and processing speed efficiency play important roles in this process. Deselection and reselection depends on the ability to suppress (deselect) newly identified task-irrelevant information as well as the ability to activate (select) newly identified task-relevant information. Efficient working memory results in material being held in working memory for a greater period of time and being increasingly available for modification. This leads to the potential for increased flexibility which in turn implies increased ability to evaluate novel solutions and consider new responses. It also suggests increased ability to select a new response to make automatic.

Therapy is cognitively demanding.

Deselection and reselection of a new process to make automatic (the process of therapy) is at first a conscious, planned, and time-consuming process. An individual who is attempting to eliminate a maladaptive, automatized process such as a complex maladaptive behavioral response or thought will struggle due to the required cognitive effort. It is likely that they will become even more inefficient and ineffective as they shift from their maladaptive strategies to newer, potentially effective but not yet automatic cognitive processes.

Learning is about connections in that what is stored together stays together in memory.

Learning new things in therapy as in all other learning occurs in context. What is learned is associated and remembered in the context of what was around it during the time it was encountered. Therefore it is critical to the process of therapy that newly learned adaptive responses should be practiced in as many new contexts as is possible. This practice should be a planned and purposeful part of treatment and not just be left to circumstance.

The basic principles of learning for NCLT are:

1. Learning is a product of working memory allocation
2. Working memory's capacity for allocation is affected by prior knowledge
3. Working memory allocation is directed by motivation

NCLT offers the following as rules that govern the process of knowledge acquisition in therapy.

How things are presented and grouped in working memory determines what procedures will be developed from their association.

If knowledge is retrieved, all other elements of knowledge to which it is connected are retrieved, and all connections between them are strengthened.

If parts of retrieved knowledge match to working memory contents, the connection between the existing knowledge and the new material are strengthened. If parts of retrieved knowledge do not match to contents in working memory, the connections are weakened and inhibited. Establishing new pattern matches (schemata) is an essential component in therapy.

If an action is successful, its connection to the knowledge of the situation in which it occurred is strengthened. If an action is unsuccessful, its connection to the knowledge of the situation in which it occurred is weakened or inhibited. The therapeutic implication of this is that new procedures must be understood and conscientiously practiced.

If knowledge has been retrieved, new information in working memory will be connected to this knowledge. This is the basis of establishing new adaptive procedures.

Any active knowledge in long-term memory is accessible to working memory.

The Goal of Therapy Is Also Competence

The term competence has been used to refer to accumulated learning experiences that result in a pattern of effective adaptation within an environment. Within the NCLT clinical context, it implies that the individual has (or lacking competence does not have) the capability to perform well in the future. Like many cognitive therapy models NCLT posits that an individual who lacks competence in an environment becomes self-aware and engages in negative self-appraisals. These negative self-appraisals are reinforced and reproduced regularly until they are automatically associated with a class of behaviors or physiological responses. NCLT theory hypothesizes that these automatically associated physiological responses and appraisals are experienced as affect states such as depression and anxiety. That is, in part, because the physiological responses associated with these affect states are also associated, through the same principles of learning, to the cognitions associated with the appraisals.

The Fourth Wave?

Given its ability to integrate most therapeutic models within its conceptual framework, it might be possible to describe NCLT as the beginning of a "fourth wave." These would be models that were able to describe the multiplicity of factors that contribute to the development of mental functioning in people, while including the ever increasing contributions of neuroscience. In addition, these models have the potential to incorporate and explain all intervention techniques under one coherent framework. This wave will have the capacity to not only conceptualize a case presentation and apply interventions, it will conceptualize a case presentation from a contextual and life course model, apply interventions specifically targeting particular schemas, and be able to teach the principles underlying both maintaining the presentation of the issues and how to impact their resolution. This wave integrates psychology and neuroscience, producing an empirically validatable and validated theory and therapy.

Index

© Springer International Publishing AG 2017
T. Wasserman, L.D. Wasserman, *Neurocognitive Learning Therapy: Theory
and Practice*, DOI 10.1007/978-3-319-60849-5